Attention Deficit Disorder Books in 1: ALL About ADHD

Thriving With Adhd Workbook + Adhd Workbook For Adults, Gain And Improve Focus, Organization, Stress Management, By Strengthening Core Skills

Gerald Paul Clifford

Thriving With ADHD Workbook

Guide to Stop Losing Focus, Impulse Control and Disorganization Through a Mind Process for a New Life

Gerald Paul Clifford

© Copyright 2020 by Gerald Paul Clifford. All right reserved.

The work contained herein has been produced with the intent to provide relevant knowledge and information on the topic on the topic described in the title for entertainment purposes only. While the author has gone to every extent to furnish up to date and true information, no claims can be made as to its accuracy or validity as the author has made no claims to be an expert on this topic. Notwithstanding, the reader is asked to do their own research and consult any subject matter experts they deem necessary to ensure the quality and accuracy of the material presented herein.

This statement is legally binding as deemed by the Committee of Publishers Association. Another body binding it legally is the American Bar Association for the territory of the United States. Other jurisdictions may apply their own legal statutes. Any reproduction, transmission, or copying of this material contained in this work without the express written consent of the copyright holder shall be deemed as a copyright violation as per the current legislation in force on the date of publishing and the subsequent time thereafter. All additional works derived from this material may be claimed by the holder of this copyright.

The data, depictions, events, descriptions, and all other information forthwith are considered to be true, fair, and accurate unless the work is expressly described as a work of fiction. Regardless of the nature of this work, the Publisher is exempt from any responsibility of actions taken by the reader in conjunction with this work. The Publisher acknowledges that the reader acts of their own accord and releases the author and Publisher of any responsibility for the observance of tips, advice, counsel, strategies, and techniques that may be offered in this volume.

Table of Contents

Introduction **8**
Chapter 1: What Is ADHD? **13**

  History of ADHD 13
  Facts and Statistics 15
  ADHD Vs. ADD 17
  Debunking Common ADHD Myths 18
  Adult ADHD 23

Chapter 2: What Are the Symptoms of ADHD? **25**

  Symptoms in Children 25

    Self-Centered 25
    Trouble Waiting 26
    Interrupting 26
    Temper Tantrums 28
    Fidgeting 28
    Tasks Left Unfinished 29
    Absence of Focus 29
    Avoidance 30
    Cannot Play Quietly 30
    Daydreaming 30
    Make Careless Mistakes 31
    Not Organized 31

  Symptoms in Adults 32

    Difficulty in Focusing 32
    Hyperfocus 33

Problems with Managing Time *33*
Disorganization *34*
Impulsiveness *34*
Forget Things Easily *35*
Hypercritical... *36*
Mood Swings *36*
Absence of Motivation *37*
Fatigue *37*
Anxiety *38*

Chapter 3: Causes of ADHD......................... 39

Can Genetics Cause ADHD? 40
How Does ADHD Affect the Brain?..................... 43
Can Pollution and Toxins Cause ADHD? 47
Other Factors That Might Lead to ADHD............. 50

Chapter 4: Diagnosis of ADHD 53

Factors That Are Looked Into............................. 54
How to Choose a Specialist for ADHD Diagnosis? 56
Diagnostic Challenges...................................... 59
Step-By-Step Guide to Diagnosing ADHD 62

Social, Academic, and Emotional Functioning Assessment *62*
Clinical Interviews.. *64*
Medical History and Physical Exam *66*

Chapter 5: Treatments for ADHD 67

What Are the Medications Used in ADHD?.......... 67

Stimulants 68

Non-Stimulants 70

Can Therapy Help? 75

Psychoeducation *75*
Behavior Therapy *75*
CBT *76*

Chapter 6: Living With ADHD 79

Binge Eating.. 79
Anxiety 83
Substance Abuse 86
Sleep Problem 87
Stress... 90

Chapter 7: How to Sharpen Your Memory When You Have ADHD? 93

What Is Working Memory? 94
When Do We Use Working Memory? 95
Tips to Boost Working Memory 98
Top Strategies for Improving Overall Memory ... 103

Chapter 8: What Should You Know About the ADHD Diet? 109

What Is ADHD Diet? 109
Sample Meal Plan 116
Best Foods for the ADHD Diet 116

Protein & Complex Carbs *117*
Vitamins & Minerals... *119*
Omega-3-Fatty Acids *120*

Chapter 9: Tips to Make Your Life More Organized 122

Throw Out What You Don't Need 122
Maintain a Planner 125
Organize Your Finances..126
Prioritize Your Happiness and Health 127
Make Decisions Within a Time Limit....................128
Don't Over-Commit 129
Your To-Do Lists Should Not Be Too Long......... 130
Limit Your Distractions 130

Chapter 10: ADHD Anger Management Tips 132

Know What Makes You Angry...............................132
Take Care of Yourself..133
Take Breaks..134
Think About the Consequences 135
Always Remain Positive..136
Learn to Express Yourself in Other Ways 137

Conclusion 139
References 143

Introduction

Congratulations on purchasing *Thriving With ADHD Workbook: Guide to Stop Losing Focus, Impulse Control and Disorganization Through a Mind Process for a New Life,* and thank you for doing so.

The following chapters will discuss every aspect of ADHD and how you can lead a productive life with it. The common symptoms in adults, who are dealing with ADHD, are irritability, chronic lateness, and impulsiveness in decisions. If you have to live with all of that for your entire life, then it can definitely be overwhelming, but in this book, you will learn how you can make it seem less of a burden. You will discover several skills that are required in an ADHD patient so that they can mitigate the symptoms and lead a better life.

Before we move into the chapters, I want to clarify something at the beginning of this book – ADHD is not the same as ADD. In previous years, when much research had not occurred on ADHD, it was known by different names, and ADD is one of them. I have given a detailed comparison between these two in Chapter 1. Even though the occurrence of this disorder was found out quite a while ago, it started occurring in greater frequency only now. The different problems that are seen, along with ADHD, include emotional and behavioral disorders and learning disabilities. They cannot spell properly or read a passage. Another thing that is seen is that ADHD is found in greater numbers in boys as compared to girls. In the beginning, it was believed that as the child grows up, the symptoms of ADHD will go away on their own, but now, researchers and psychiatrists understand the fact that ADHD is not a temporary condition but a lifelong one. The symptoms can definitely be managed, but they still persist in some form or the other in adulthood.

There are several proven strategies and mental tools mentioned in this book that will not only help you navigate your life but also improve your management skills. If you are someone who is dealing with ADHD yourself or if you have a family member who has this problem, then this book will help you in several ways moving forward. Building the life that you always wanted will seem possible now that you have the required skillset.

People are not only beginning to understand this problem better, but there have been several advances in terms of treatment of this disorder. In this book, I aim to give my audience a better understanding of how ADHD affects the life of a person and how these symptoms can be managed with a little bit of effort.

But I want to stress on the fact that you should not consider this book as a substitute for seeking proper treatment. This book is more of an aid to the diagnosis and line of treatment followed by a certified physician. I am sure by the end of this book, I will be able to answer several questions that pop up in people's minds.

People who suffer from ADHD not only have to deal with several behavioral problems but also learning disabilities. All of these symptoms together make up the problem of ADHD. If someone is facing only learning difficulties, it might not be due to ADHD. Also, you have to keep in mind that both these classes of symptoms have to be dealt with differently because the strategies you need to manage behavioral symptoms is not the same as learning difficulties.

In this book, you will get a summary of all the things that humankind has learned about ADHD so far. Apart from that, you will also get detailed information on various aspects of ADHD, as collected from several medical researches and reports. The symptoms of ADHD, as seen in children, are not the same when these same people move into adulthood. I will discuss the symptoms of both children and adults separately.

Some of the very important points that will be elaborated in this book are as follows –

- In the childhood years, ADHD is a very serious mental health disorder and is often overlooked. According to statistics, the disorder is more commonly seen in boys than that in girls.

- ADHD does not cure by itself when a child moves into adulthood. The symptoms might manifest themselves in a different way, but the disorder itself is carried on. It is a lifelong problem.

- It has been found that ADHD is genetic. Concrete evidence to the causes of ADHD has not been found, and it has not been found out clearly as to how this disorder is passed, but the chemical composition of the brain is altered.

- There are several other disorders that co-exist with ADHD, and this makes the diagnosis of the problem quite confusing. People might have behavioral and learning disorders, along with having ADHD.

- The proper diagnosis of ADHD is important if you want the person to recover and lead a normal life. Diagnosis in the childhood years makes adulthood easier because the child learns the coping strategies in the early years, and by the time they are adults, they become an expert at managing their symptoms. The earlier the treatment is provided to a person, the lesser is the chance of the behavioral problems going out of hand.

- There are no laboratory or psychological examinations that help in finding out whether a child has ADHD or not. The method of diagnosis is solely based on a series of conversations and other achievement and IQ tests.

- Proper medication really proves to be helpful in the case of ADHD because they help in lowering the effect of the symptoms. Another thing to keep in mind is that the medicines that are prescribed in ADHD do not have any addictive effect on the patients. Apart from medicines, behavioral therapy should also be done. When an ADHD patient moves into adulthood, other therapies like psychoeducational therapy and couple therapy provide effective results.

I am thankful to you for choosing this book out of the several options in the market. I tried my best to make this as informative as possible, and so I sincerely hope that you enjoy it.

Chapter 1: What Is ADHD?

This is an introductory chapter that will give you the basic concepts of ADHD that you need to know before proceeding to the later chapters of this book. ADHD is an acronym for Attention Deficit Hyperactivity Disorder. As the term suggests, people who have ADHD show impulsive behaviors and are abnormally hyperactive. It is primarily a mental health disorder, and people who experience this cannot sit in one place for too long and cannot focus on the tasks that they are doing. Awareness about this disorder will help people understand it better and seek the help they need. With proper medication and therapy, ADHD can be managed even though it cannot be cured.

History of ADHD

Children are the ones who are most commonly diagnosed with ADHD. It is also referred to as a neurodevelopmental disorder. The age of 7 is when most children are diagnosed with this problem. Another common feature that has been noticed is that it is the boys who are more commonly seen to have this problem as compared to girls. Symptoms might be noticeable in adults as well. Initially, ADHD was not referred to by this term but by a different term – hyperkinetic impulse disorder. After that, it was classified under the umbrella term of mental disorder by the APA or American Psychiatric Association towards the latter part of the 1960s.

Here is a brief description of the timeline of this disease that will help you understand the history better –

- It was in the year 1902 that ADHD was mentioned for the first time. At that time, it was only defined as a defect in children that affects their moral control and is rather abnormal, and this description was given by Sir George Still, who was a pediatrician.

- Then, it was in 1936 when Benzedrine was approved by the FDA. But immediately in the next year, the medicine was found to display some side effects. When this medicine was given to children, their performance and behavior in school showed considerable improvement. However, these findings were largely ignored at that time.

- In the first edition of the DSM, ADHD was not even recognized in the category of mental disorder. The first edition was published in the year 1952. Then in the year 1968, a second edition was published, and in this one, hyperkinetic impulse disorder was listed.

- By 1955, people started understanding ADHD and its nature, and the drug Ritalin was approved by the FDA. This drug is used even today.

- In 1980 came the third edition of the DSM, and it was here that the term ADD or attention deficit disorder was used for the first time in place of hyperkinetic impulse disorder. Two subtypes of ADD were formed because of this list, and they were – ADD without hyperactivity and ADD with hyperactivity.

- Finally, in the year 1987, a revised version was published, and here the term ADHD was used

- Then, in the year 2000, the DSM was released as a fourth edition which also identified three subtypes of ADHD, namely –

    o Predominantly inattentive type ADHD

    o Combined type ADHD

    o Predominantly hyperactive-impulse type ADHD

Facts and Statistics

Before we move into greater details, here are five quick facts about ADHD that everyone should know –

- In a person's lifetime, 4.2% of women are usually diagnosed with ADHD. But the numbers are quite high in men at 13%.

- As compared to women, men are most likely to develop symptoms of ADHD. In fact, there are three times more chances of men developing ADHD than women.

- There is no hard and fast rule that ADHD will happen only in childhood. People in America deal with ADHD even in their adulthood, and statistics show that it is almost 4% of adults who are above the age of 18 that encounter ADHD.

- At an average, people are diagnosed with ADHD at the age of 7.

- It is between the ages of three and six that the symptoms of ADHD first start to appear.

Now, here are some other important facts that you should know about –

- All the races are affected by ADHD. However, in the span of 2001-2010, a sudden surge of ADHD was noticed in black girls of non-Hispanic origin, and there was as much as over 90% increase.

- 5.5% of Latino children are affected with ADHD, 9.5% of Black children are affected, and 9.8% of White children are affected.

- About 6.4 million children in America have been diagnosed with this disorder. They are all between the ages of 4 and 17.

- Even though the numbers differ from state to state – about 6.1 % of children in America are under ADHD medication and receiving treatment. But 23% of children in American are not receiving any kind of counseling or medication for ADHD.

ADHD Vs. ADD

You will often see these two terms being used on the internet, but here is something that most people miss – ADHD and ADD are not the same things. They are two different problems. If you read the History of ADHD section in this chapter, then you will know that ADD is basically an older term. In fact, previously, people did not recognize ADHD as a separate entity, and ADD was used to refer to everything. For decades, no proper diagnosis was made.

The main difference between these two terms lies in the symptoms. The three major symptoms of ADHD are as follows –

- Hyperactivity
- Inattentiveness
- Impulsivity

People who are suffering from ADHD struggle with all the three symptoms, but in some people, trouble focusing is the major problem. These people would have been put in the category of ADD if it was before the year 1994, but today, the diagnosis would be made as ADHD. This type of ADHD is described or referred to by several other terms as well, some of which are inattentive ADHD, ADHD inattentive type, or ADHD without hyperactivity. But the common factor in all of these terms is inattention being the main symptom. You will learn more about the various symptoms of ADHD in Chapter 2.

Debunking Common ADHD Myths

Just like everything else, there are some common myths about ADHD in everyone's minds, and I am going to clear the air in this section. These misconceptions need to be cleared; otherwise, those who are present in the community will be the ones affected the most. Moreover, these myths are why people cannot access proper treatment or diagnosis on time or worse – they are often misunderstood. So, I really hope this section is going to be helpful to all of you.

- ***Girls cannot get ADHD*** – This is absolutely a myth because girls do get ADHD. But the origin of this myth lies in the fact that signs of hyperactivity in young girls are not often seen compared to boys in whom these signs are so prevalent. So, due to the lack of prominent behavioral issues in young girls, people often think that girls cannot get ADHD and so they are also not evaluated as much as boys. Also, the major consequence of this myth is that the condition of ADHD in girls keeps progressing because most of them are left untreated, and so as they grow up, they face issues like anxiety, mood swings, an antisocial personality, and when they approach adulthood, they face other comorbid disorders as well. So, boys and girls should be treated in the same way when it comes to ADHD; otherwise, we won't be able to provide them with the care and support they deserve and need.

- ***Laziness is a sign of ADHD*** – When people are diagnosed with ADHD, several of them are scolded or taunted for being lazy and this, in turn, leads them to feel bad or guilty about themselves. They constantly keep comparing themselves to others because they do not feel productive enough. They see others and want to feel motivated just like everyone else, but they can't. A sustained mental effort is very important in people with ADHD to help them get the day-to-day things done. They have to be reminded constantly because disorganization in life is a very common symptom of ADHD, and we are going to address this issue in this book. But this doesn't mean that they are lazy. They also want to achieve great things in life, but the effort required by an ADHD person to complete a simple task is way more than anyone else. In fact, answering an email might seem too difficult because they have to focus on it for a certain period of time to compose a reply. But do you know why this myth is so harmful? This myth creates a sense of failure and disappointment in those who are suffering from ADHD. They lose their confidence, and their self-esteem takes a direct hit.

- ***ADHD is the result of bad parenting*** – You will often see the parents of ADHD kids and adults blaming themselves because they think it is their bad parenting that resulted in the problem. But it is not. It is true that when someone is diagnosed with ADHD, a certain structure is necessary for their lives, but if the parents think that scolding their child or blurting out harsh words would solve the problem, it won't. In fact, it can make things worse. ADHD needs to be treated just like any other health problem. It needs medication and psychotherapy.

- ***ADHD is not a serious problem*** – Many people think that ADHD is not a serious problem and so they don't take the appropriate measures. I will agree with the fact that this mental health problem is not life-threatening, but that doesn't mean you will not get bothered by it. The quality of life of a person is severely impacted when they are diagnosed with ADHD. Substance use disorders and anxiety are two things that come hand-in-hand with the problem. Moreover, even adults need to be constantly reminded of their responsibilities so that they can keep up with their lives. These people have to put in a lot of effort to stay financially stable, and they are almost paranoid at all times because their inattentiveness might cost them their jobs. Even though some measures are taken in educational institutions to accommodate people with ADHD, but when it comes to a work setting, employers are not really willing to cooperate with any delay.

- ***ADHD is not a real health issue*** – This point is also similar to the one we just discussed where ADHD is not taken seriously but here, we take things a step further and deal with the myth where people think that there are no chemical imbalanced in the body due to ADHD. But this is not true because all the important brain chemicals like norepinephrine, dopamine, and glutamate change their functioning in people with ADHD, and that is why medication is necessary.

- ***ADHD happens only in children*** – It is true that ADHD is common in children, but when a child is not diagnosed properly, then ADHD is carried onto adulthood. If they are diagnosed with ADHD for the first time when they are adults, it means that they were not diagnosed before. And once they are diagnosed, they will be able to realize that they did have the symptoms in their childhood years, but no one paid heed to them. Moreover, some people may be diagnosed in their childhood, but as they grow up, the symptoms of ADHD might not remain the same and evolve into something different.

- ***ADHD can be cured with the help of medication*** – People often have this misconception that just because they are taking meds for ADHD, it is going to cure them. But that's not how it works. Medication for ADHD does not cure the problem. Instead, it simply helps the person to cope with the symptoms. I hate to break it down to you, but ADHD is a lifelong condition and a chronic one at that. The only thing that makes life easier is by learning different skills and coping strategies. Throughout their lives, they will keep on building several such new skills and keep taking medication to aid the process.

- ***ADHD is a type of learning disability*** – This myth itself is the reason why so many people are misdiagnosed. Learning disabilities are completely different, and ADHD is not one of those. It is true that the symptoms of ADHD can hamper learning by lowering the capability to focus. Moreover, in some people, ADHD and learning disabilities co-exist, which makes diagnosis all the more confusing and also leads to this myth being so popular.

- ***Kids will outgrow ADHD*** – You cannot outgrow ADHD. It doesn't happen like that. The development changes in the body of a person and changes in brain composition can alter the symptoms a bit, but ADHD, at the end of the day, is a lifelong condition.

These myths need to be dispelled because it is because of these misconceptions that there is a delay in proper diagnosis, and society doesn't take appropriate measures to accommodate people with ADHD. Since there are no visible symptoms of this disorder, people often misjudge it or misdiagnose it. This is because people do not have any idea as to what they are talking about. And on top of everything, the misconceptions only add to the shame and guilt of the patients. So, accurate diagnosis is very important.

Adult ADHD

Whenever we talk about ADHD, the first image that pops up in our minds is that of a seven-year-old kid who doesn't concentrate at school and keeps running around the house. But people are oblivious to the fact that adults, too, are affected by ADHD, and it amounts to as much as 4% of Americans. In adults, however, the symptom of hyperactivity is not so much prevalent or common as in kids. But even then, adults face a lot of problems in their personal and professional lives because of ADHD. It also severely affects their social interactions.

We will discuss the symptoms in detail in the next chapter, but something that you have to understand is that ADHD does not show itself in the same in adults as in children. That is why so many adults either go undiagnosed or are misdiagnosed. In the case of adult ADHD, all the complex tasks of day-to-day life are hampered, and this includes decision-making, judgments, memory, and initiative. Two of the problems that are often confused with ADHD are depression and anxiety attacks. The reason behind this is the similarity in symptoms.

Whenever an adult is diagnosed with ADHD, you have to understand that the person had ADHD even when they were children. It was either not diagnosed at all due to a lack of proper resources, or it was misdiagnosed as a learning disability. In some cases, these people did not have serious symptoms in their childhood, and that is why they were not diagnosed. Whatever the reason may be, since the problem was not diagnosed as ADHD, it did not receive the treatment it should have.

Chapter 2: What Are the Symptoms of ADHD?

In this chapter, we are going to talk about the symptoms of ADHD and how it looks in both adults and children. Keep in mind that most of the time, the symptoms vary so much from one person to another that it becomes very difficult to identify ADHD. Some people display elaborate symptoms, while others might show only a few symptoms.

Symptoms in Children

In the first section, we will go through the various symptoms as observed in a child.

Self-Centered

The first symptom of ADHD is that the child often does not show any type of empathy towards others and does not try to understand what other people are going through. They cannot understand the needs of others, and thus, they come across as self-centered. This symptom itself leads to other symptoms, mainly trouble to wait and to interrupt often. But are they really self-centered? Maybe not because most of the notion about ADHD kids being self-centered comes from the fact that they are always involved in extreme self-care. They have a routine that they follow rigidly, and this means they do exercise daily, eat at a specific time, and go to bed early. But all of these things help them handle the condition in a better way, but not everyone can see it this way. Moreover, the communication skills of ADHD kids are very poor, and this is also the reason why they come off as self-centered.

Trouble Waiting

The next symptom that we are going to discuss is quite a common one – ADHD kids can never hold the patience of waiting for their turn. This applies to any situation where they have to wait in line. Moreover, if they are asked to wait until someone comes back, even then, they cannot sit in one place and will keep fidgeting.

Interrupting

This symptom can be very annoying because ADHD kids do not understand when they shouldn't speak up and when they should. Suppose there is a conversation happening which does not involve them, they might suddenly speak up, interrupting the conversation. Similarly, if other children are playing games that don't involve them, the ADHD kids might go and interrupt their game. But there are several strategies that can help your child practice self-control. The important thing to understand here is that children with ADHD do not mean any harm, and they do not interrupt willingly. Most of the time, they do not even realize that they are interrupting. And this is mainly because the ADHD kids do not understand when someone is angry with them or even frowning.

Temper Tantrums

A very common symptom of ADHD in kids is their temper flare-ups. In fact, anger and ADHD really go hand-in-hand. The reason behind this is that children who are suffering from ADHD get stressed even in the most commonplace of situations. And so, they are not able to keep a check on their emotions. You will often notice them having an anger outburst in the most inappropriate situation of all. Also, anyone who has ADHD is already very emotionally sensitive. When the kids go to school, they might have some negative experiences as they are not like the other kids. And as parents, you might not always hear about these experiences your kids have at school. When the child comes back home, they have even more tasks to complete apart from the stress that is already on their minds. So, it is quite natural for the kid to show a temper tantrum because he/she is already quite overwhelmed.

Fidgeting

Fidgeting is related to the hyperactivity factor of ADHD. Whenever a child keeps making restless movements, they are said to have bouts of fidgeting, which is a very common symptom indeed. But parents need to understand that the child is not doing this on purpose. The fidgeting is out of their control, and it usually shows that the child is nervous or under stress, or simply bored. You will also notice your child fidgeting when you ask them to sit in one place for too long.

Tasks Left Unfinished

You will often find that a child who has ADHD is interested in doing a lot of things, but the problem is, they are not too much inclined towards finishing what they started. Let us say your child has a ton of homework to do, and she starts doing it in the evening. But before she can complete it, she hops on to some other task or starts playing. For others, this might seem a problem that is easy to solve and that the child is doing this because they are not trying hard to focus. But that's not the problem here. The child slowly becomes the jack-of-all-trades, and yet they cannot master any. This even applies to leisure activities. If a child with ADHD starts watching a particular cartoon series, then the chances are that they are not going to finish it and would soon start doing something else.

Absence of Focus

Lack of focus is a symptom of ADHD in children, and it affects every aspect of their lives. Even if you are talking to an ADHD child directly, they might not be able to pay you the attention that is required. When you ask them to repeat what you have just said, it is highly likely that they won't be able to do that because they were not focusing on what you were saying. But here you should remind yourself that not every problem that has an attention deficit symptoms is ADHD. But if your child is experiencing troubles in focusing, then the best way to find that out is through the performance of the child in school. Shorter spans of attention are what cause the absence of focus.

Avoidance

All the above symptoms that I have mentioned above leads to a type of avoidance in a kid suffering from ADHD. The kids tend to avoid anything that needs them to wait, focus, or give a sustained mental effort. This includes a lot of things and almost all types of schoolwork. For teenagers, this can also mean household chores, which require extensive physical exertion. Anything that requires cognitive effort is totally off the list when it comes to people with ADHD.

Cannot Play Quietly

ADHD children have the habit of talking excessively, and so they are not able to play quietly. This symptom is also a result of the fidgeting problem. ADHD kids are not inclined towards activities and games that require them to stay quiet for a certain period of time. They are always impatient and have this constant need to move around.

Daydreaming

This is another of the very common symptoms of children who have ADHD. You have to keep in mind that daydreaming is just one of the symptoms of ADHD. You cannot diagnose someone with ADHD just because they were daydreaming because lots of kids do. Daydreaming along is never enough to conclude that a child is suffering from ADHD. But those who do have ADHD and daydream are often found staring out in the distance and lost in their own world. They are not even much involved in playing with other kids.

Make Careless Mistakes

Children with ADHD need to be constantly reminded and guided to help them complete their tasks, and even after all of that, they make mistakes that are rather careless. Even if you make a set of instructions for the kid, you will notice that the child is facing problems following those instructions. But just because they are making mistakes doesn't mean they are lazy or do not have the willingness to fulfill their dreams. Kids with ADHD have a tendency to make silly mistakes in subjects like Maths, which might seem rather easy to others.

Not Organized

Being organized is a skill that is required at every age, but with ADHD, staying organized is probably the biggest struggle. This can be noticed even at a young age. Kids often fail to keep track of their activities and tasks. The assignments and projects keep piling up, and prioritizing is something that ADHD kids have trouble with. They have to be constantly kept on a routine by their parents, and by following different strategies since childhood, ADHD becomes manageable by the time these kids become adults.

These were some of the common symptoms that are noticed in ADHD kids, but as the children grow up, you will notice that these kids are often seen to be immature when compared to others of their age. They have trouble with so many aspects of daily life like driving, managing time, compromise, understanding social cues, and so on.

Symptoms in Adults

When ADHD is diagnosed and treated since childhood years, it becomes easier to manage when they grow up. But at other times, the symptoms go unnoticed, and ADHD is left undiagnosed. It doesn't receive appropriate treatment at the right time, and thus, symptoms put a strain on the everyday aspects of life. In order to ensure proper management of the problem, identifying the symptoms and seeking help from a doctor is mandatory. In this section, I am going to introduce you to some of the common symptoms of ADHD, as seen in adults.

Difficulty in Focusing

One of the most prominent signs of ADHD in adults is the inability to focus. Adults with ADHD cannot seem to concentrate on anything for too long. They are distracted very easily, and even when they are in the middle of a conversation, they find it really hard to keep listening to someone over an extended period of time or make an effort to carry on the conversation. Another sign of difficulty in focusing is when a person misses out important details from a conversation and is not able to keep up with their deadlines. In this book, you will learn about several strategies that you can use to increase your focusing power.

Hyperfocus

In the previous section, we talked about the difficulties faced by people when it comes to focusing, but the flip side to that is also common in adult ADHD, and that is known as hyperfocus. As you might have guessed from the term, hyper-focusing is a state when the person is so engrossed in the task they are doing that they are simply not willing to look in any other direction. They zero in on that single task with a lot of intensity, and you can also say that it is completely opposite to that of distractibility. People don't even realize how hours have passed by, and they were fixated on that one single task.

Problems with Managing Time

This is another trait of adults suffering from ADHD. They cannot figure out how they can effectively spend their time and complete all the tasks on their to-do list. You will often find people with ADHD procrastinating or consistently missing out on appointments. Some people even forget invitations to parties and weddings. The reaction to time and the perception of time in people with ADHD is quite different from those of others. In simpler words, their thought on the time needed to do a particular task might not be the same as someone else's. Some of the researchers and experts have come up with a special term 'time blindness,' which points to this problem of managing time. And the fact that ADHD makes them easy prey to distraction makes matters worse when it comes to managing time.

Disorganization

People will ADHD feel that their life is chaotic, and even when they have a routine in place, things are not quite organized. They might constantly be searching for that one pair of socks that seem to get lost every other day. They fall behind on their monthly bills. Or, their work desk is always full of clutter. In extreme cases, people also lose their jobs, or their careers suffer just because of their disorganized behavior. They constantly feel exhaustion and are overwhelmed with the growing burden of work that is left unfinished. However, if proper strategies are undertaken, these symptoms can be managed. Every person's needs in the case of ADHD are different, and so careful assessment has to be done regarding which strategies you should use.

Impulsiveness

Now we come to the symptom of impulsivity, which means that adults who are suffering from ADHD take actions before thinking them through. There are multiple ways in which this particular symptom can manifest itself in a person. Also, it is not the same in everyone. Something may be true for you, but it might not be the same for someone else. Some common ways in which this symptom shows itself are – finishing tasks in a rush, doing things or saying stuff that is considered to be inappropriate in social settings, interrupting an important conversation suddenly, and doing things without giving a thought to the gravity of the consequences that are to follow. One of the best ways to identify whether a person is impulsive or not is to have a close look at their shopping habits. If a person consistently buys things that he/she hardly needs or even cannot afford in normal situations, then they are making impulsive decisions. It is one of the symptoms pointing in the direction of ADHD. It is because of this symptom of impulsivity that adults with ADHD also have temper outbursts from time to time.

Forget Things Easily

People are quite confused about this symptom because all of us tend to forget things from time to time, but does that mean we all have ADHD? No. But on the other hand, those who have ADHD also show symptoms of forgetfulness. They keep searching for common things like keys or glasses because they keep misplacing them. They can even miss their medical appointments or forget to call back people. The bottom line of all this is that whether forgetfulness is due to ADHD or not, it has quite damaging consequences on people's lives and also harms relationships. The forgetfulness in ADHD adults becomes scary when they have important responsibilities like looking after a child. There have been cases where the parent forgot to pick the child up from school or dance lessons.

Hypercritical

The sense of self-image in adults with ADHD is very bad, and they are very much hypercritical. The main reason behind this is that they are so burdened by the disappointments of not completing work on time or meeting several other personal failures that their self-esteem suffers. They start criticizing themselves for even the smallest mistakes. They no longer see things positively, and everything is in a negative light. So, everything starting from impulsiveness to difficulty in focusing contributes to the problem of being hypercritical.

Mood Swings

Adults who have ADHD are quite emotionally unstable. All of us experience impatience and anxiety in our lives, which also manifests themselves in the form of anger. But these emotions are magnified to a greater level in those who are suffering from ADHD. These mood swings also affect their jobs and personal lives. Gradually, they feel demoralized, and as if they can do nothing with the situation. Dealing with ADHD symptoms in life is already a difficult task, and there are numerous challenges that crop up along the way, and so, life, in general, becomes chaotic. When these emotional problems are not tended to, they start accumulating until a final outburst and wreaks havoc in life.

Absence of Motivation

Adults with ADHD often don't feel motivated to do things like others. The root of this problem lies in the fact that these people are not able to focus, and thus, they feel unmotivated to complete the task. Moreover, as you already know, the feeling of being overwhelmed is very common in ADHD adults, and this adds to the feeling of being unmotivated. Most people don't even try to accomplish a task and give up way before that. They can't seem to figure out what the right path is in order to go from one point to another. They cannot stay fixated to one thing at a time and jump from one task to another. In this way, nothing is ever completed.

Fatigue

People often overlook the fact that one of the most important symptoms of ADHD is fatigue. I know that you might be surprised by this revelation, but this is actually true, and there are multiple reasons behind this. Firstly, those with ADHD are hyperactive most of the time, and this makes them feel tired. They also suffer from inconsistent sleeping patterns. Secondly, in some people, fatigue results from the constant struggle that they have to engage in to focus on their day-to-day tasks. And thirdly, another reason is the medications prescribed for ADHD, which also makes people feel like they are tired all the time. No matter what the cause is, the main point is that fatigue is a very difficult thing to deal with, and it can make life worse.

Anxiety

I have referred to this term quite a lot in this chapter, but you also need to be aware of the fact that anxiety, in fact, is a direct sign of ADHD as well. People feel that they just keep thinking all the time, and there is no moment of peace in their lives. They get frustrated because they have to keep fighting this constant need to keep moving. This is also the reason why people with ADHD are so restless. Another reason why people get so anxious when they have ADHD is that they forget important things. When they cannot remember stuff, it makes them anxious. Moreover, those who are facing sleep problems have to go through even worse situations.

All of the symptoms of ADHD in adults mentioned in this chapter give rise to several personal and professional problems. But these difficulties can be overcome, and you will learn to do that in the latter part of this book. If you want to read about why ADHD happens, the next chapter will give you a lot of information on that.

Chapter 3: Causes of ADHD

All the scientific research that has been done until now has confirmed that ADHD is a disorder that affects the brain. In this chapter, you will see how at its very core, a problem in brain development that is passed on genetically is the root cause of this disorder. Most of the cases of ADHD that are brought to light have one thing in common – the brain structure is abnormal, and this happens in the unborn child and manifests itself in different ways once the child is born. Some other things that are noticed include an imbalance in the chemical functioning of the brain, and the messages in the brain are not relayed properly. Another thing worth noticing in al of this is that the drugs that are used in the treatment of ADHD are very effective. They can even minimize the effect of the symptoms on the body and corrects many of the imbalances.

The seriousness of the problem can be handled and managed only if the diagnosis of ADHD is made at the right moment, and appropriate measures have been taken. Bad parenting is never the cause of ADHD, and we have clarified this myth before, but what you need to learn is that sometimes, some parents do not bring up their ADHD kids attending to their special needs, and this is what makes situations worse. In the same way, if the parents follow all the strategies for coping up, things will be better for the child when he/she grows up to be an adult. Having said that, I want to say it again that no matter how bad your parenting is, even if you have abused your child, you cannot say that your child got ADHD because of it since it does not spread like that. The child or the person who has been suddenly diagnosed with ADHD was definitely predisposed to the disorder. The seriousness of the ADHD symptoms is affected to some extent by the techniques used by parents during their upbringing. But this does not mean that parental approaches somehow cause ADHD. ADHD is solely biological, and the management of the symptoms becomes easier with these psychological approaches.

Before we go into the different causes behind ADHD, I want to make one point clear, and that is – no one is sure as to what is the exact cause behind this disorder. What people have found out until now is that there are multiple possible reasons behind it, and these reasons might not be the same in everyone. For someone, it might be the genes, whereas, for others, it might be something else. Several assessments of behaviors have been done over the years to improve the understanding of this disorder. The heritability factor has received quite an attention after several researchers providing evidence through their assessments. It has been noticed that the genetic contribution is quite popular in those who are being diagnosed with ADHD.

Can Genetics Cause ADHD?

In this section, we are going to approach the issue of whether ADHD is caused by genetic factors or not. Well, in several cases, it has been seen that there is strong evidence of genetics playing a role in causing ADHD. If a family member already has ADHD, then a particular person is already prone to developing it as much as four times higher than anyone else. Several genes are now being investigated by scientists all over the world to find a strong and definite connection with ADHD. The genes that are closely related to dopamine are the ones that are most commonly investigated. This is because a common trait is found in people with ADHD – their dopamine levels are way lower than others who don't have ADHD. Here is a quick fact that you should be aware of – dopamine is a chemical in the brain whose main function is to help a person concentrate on something consistently and regularly. But you should be aware of the myths about ADHD since they tend to outnumber the facts and often guide you in the wrong direction.

In short, even though the researchers have not been able to pinpoint any particular cause for ADHD, they definitely have narrowed down to a number of things that are probably behind it, and genetics is one of them. When brain imaging was done of the patients, it revealed that there were significant differences with those who do not have ADHD. Thus, the cause of ADHD is completely biological, and it is not caused by consuming too much sugar or bad parenting or any other hoax that you heard from your neighbor.

In fact, it has also been noticed in studies that the parts of the brain which are responsible for helping you to concentrate often have thinner tissues in patients with ADHD, and this is also correlated to the presence of a particular gene. This gene, when investigated, showed that these changes are temporary. When a child approached adolescence and then adulthood, the brain tissues also undergo developmental changes, and thus, several symptoms either manifest themselves differently or subside.

So, it can be said that in some families, ADHD is definitely passed down from parents to children, and this is reinforced by the fact that 1/3rd of those fathers who were diagnosed with ADHD in their childhood years have a child who also has ADHD. Another evidence that suggests the presence of a link between genetics and ADHD is that the disorder is present in most of the identical twins. Also, since ADHD is not a simple disorder and involves a lot of complex aspects, scientists believe that it is not regulated by only one gene but rather two. As far as the genetic field is concerned, there is a lot left to do to find a piece of solid evidence. But if and when this link is found, it would be of immense help to the specialists to diagnose ADHD, and this, in turn, would help the patients to receive the right line of treatment from an early stage. In fact, since the symptoms vary from one person to another, concrete evidence linking a gene can even make the treatment process easier. An Australian study has even shown evidence that when it comes to identical twins, the risk of developing

ADHD is even greater as compared to singletons (Megan R. McDougall, 2006).

Another study has also proven that genetics does have a serious role to play when it comes to ADHD. In 2010, children with ADHD were examined, and it was found that the brains of these kids either had duplicated pieces of a certain DNA or completely missing DNA (Nigel M. Williams, 2010). The genetic segments that were studied in this experiment are also speculated to be linked with schizophrenia and autism.

How Does ADHD Affect the Brain?

I have already mentioned earlier that ADHD affects the brain, and in this section, we are going to see how. There are several functional and structural differences spotted in the brain of an ADHD patient. When neuro-imaging of an ADHD brain was performed, it showed that the rate of maturation of the brain is much slower. So, kids who do not have ADHD mature faster than those who have ADHD. Apart from this, the areas of the brain that are responsible for playing a part in ADHD symptoms also show some structural differences, and this has been proven by recent research. According to research, a 5% reduction in size is noticed in some regions of the brain of ADHD patients, namely – basal ganglia, striatum, prefrontal cortex, and cerebellum (Ajay Singh, 2015). Now this structural difference that I have mentioned has been found to be consistent in the patients with ADHD, but this is not enough for the proper diagnosis of any random individual.

However, I hope that one day all of these imaging studies and their findings might lead to the discovery of some technique that will help in the diagnosis of ADHD. But if we are talking about today, then this is still a controversial matter.

Apart from this, there are also several chemical changes that are observed in the brain in a patient who is suffering from attention-deficit hyperactivity disorder. As far as the mental health disorders are concerned, you would be surprised to know that ADHD is, in fact, one of the initial disorders that were related to the reduced amounts of dopamine (an important neurotransmitter). ADHD was also one of the first mental health disorders that actually responded positively to the medicines that were used to treat the deficiency of dopamine. When ADHD is diagnosed in adults or even children, it is found that their levels of dopamine are quite low.

The neurotransmitter activity is gravely affected in four core regions of the brain in ADHD patients, and these functional areas are as follows –

- **Frontal Cortex** – Everything staring from executing something to organizing stuff and maintaining concentration is maintained by the frontal cortex region. Inattention is often caused by a reduction in levels of dopamine in this part of the brain. The executive functions are also affected, and so is the ability to organize.

- **Basal Ganglia** – Next, we come to that region of the brain, which is mainly responsible for maintaining proper communication between different parts. The basal ganglia can be called a neural circuit in simple terms. Whenever a part of the brain has to relay information to another part, it first comes to the basal ganglia. From there, it is then sent to that part of the brain which needs to be communicated. But when the basal ganglia do not have adequate levels of dopamine, it undergoes a phase that is often referred to as the 'short circuit,' and this is what causes impulsiveness and loss of attention.

- **Limbic System** – Contrary to the other parts, the limbic system is situated in the depths of the human brain, and its main function is the manifestation of emotions. When dopamine is deficient in this region, emotions are no longer stable, and the person suffers from restlessness and loss of attention.

- **Reticular Activating System** – There are more than one pathways in your brain, and one of the most critical relay systems is the reticular activating system. And if this system faces any deficiency in the levels of dopamine, then the instant result is hyperactivity, impulsivity, and inattention.

You also have to keep in mind that proper functioning of the brain is only possible when all of these parts of the brain interact with one another to work in a synchronized fashion. But a dopamine deficiency prevents that from happening. So, even if one among these four regions or all four regions has a problem with dopamine, then ADHD might occur. There is, however, no concrete proof regarding which part of the brain is responsible for ADHD symptoms. More clinical trials and experience are required to say anything specifically. The quality of ADHD treatment will improve only when the understanding of these neurochemicals increases.

NAMI or National Institue of Mental Health had published a study in which they were able to pinpoint a particular part of the brain that is affected by ADHD (Philip Shaw, 2007). The part of the brain that is responsible for helping you stay attentive displays thinner tissues in those who have ADHD. But the study also concluded something positive, and that is – when the children grow up, in some of them, the thinner tissues became normal. And consequently, with an increase in the thickness of the tissues, the symptoms of ADHD also began to subside.

Another observation that has been made so far by scientists is that in a small percentage of children, ADHD shows itself after a brain injury. The injury might be a physical one or even an increased exposure to harmful chemicals (you are going to learn more about that in the next section). Experts have noted that people who were not affected by ADHD previously developed the symptoms after encountering head injuries. It is possibly because of damage caused to the frontal lobe. It is also the reason why the frontal lobe of the human brain is so extensively researched with respect to ADHD.

Can Pollution and Toxins Cause ADHD?

A scientific research was conducted to find out whether there is a link between disorders like autism and ADHD with that of being exposed to everyday chemicals. The research showed that some kind of link is present and that chemicals in toothpaste or other products related to personal care, cleaning products, flooring, and even foods can contribute to causing ADHD. Moreover, the various systems in our body are still in the stage of development when we are infants, and that is when the human is most vulnerable to these chemicals. The overall physical health of the child and its brain can have a lifelong impact if serious toxins are exposed to important regions of the body when the baby is in a fetal stage. These toxins are known to negatively affect the course of normal brain development in children.

A report was launched by the LDDI or the Learning and Developmental Disabilities Initiative regarding the fact that learning disabilities in humans can occur as a result of certain toxic chemicals. This report was published in the year 2010. In this report, it has been mentioned that people are affected by chemicals even if they are not living somewhere that is right next to a dumping yard or factory. We are exposed to harmful chemicals on an everyday basis in the most commonplace areas, and these chemicals have the ability to damage the brain. And here are some of those common chemicals that are harmful –

- Do you know what materials like Scotchgard and Teflon are made of? They contain a particular type of chemical known as PFC or perfluorinated compounds. The main function of these compounds is that they do not allow the food to stick to pans, cooking utensils, carpets, or even curtains.

- Next, we come to another range of harmful chemicals that are easily found in household chemicals, and these are – PBDEs or polybrominated diphenyl ethers. They are found in bedding, furniture, and even clothing items. Their main function is that of a fire retardant.

- The third compound on this list is something that you will get in your personal care products – triclosan. It is found in toothpaste and soaps, and many other items as well. It protects you from harmful bacteria and is itself a harmful chemical.

- The next chemical that I am going to name is already very well-known as being harmful – phthalates. They help to make things pliable and soft, and they are present in a lot of rubber-based and plastic materials like raincoats, bottles, toys, and so on. You will also get them in shampoos and soaps.

- Lastly, BPA or Bisphenol A is another chemical that you should be aware of. It is present in several containers and even food cans, and it is mainly an epoxy resin. Those plastic containers you use at home often contain BPA, and they are even found in certain products made from paper. However, these days you will get several alternative options that are BPA-free.

The participants in the initiative made by LDDI were tested for these toxins. There were a total of 89 chemicals that were studied. Every participant in that listed tested positive for at least twenty-six of those harmful chemicals. Scary, isn't it?

A study was performed by the University of Calgary in 2015 that found that some zebrafish were hyperactive, and this symptom could be traced back to chemicals like BPA and BPS, both of which are present in plastic. But did you know that zebrafish is very important in the studies of embryonic brain development of humans? Yes, and the main reason behind this is that about 4/5th of the genes are common between humans and zebrafish. Moreover, the processes and stages of development are also similar. Since BPS and BPA exposure to these fishes showed negative results in terms of brain developments, the findings of the study proved to be a smoking gun.

Another study that was conducted in the year 2015 showed that ADHD could also be caused by increased exposure to lead (Joel T. Nigg, 2015). But the researchers had also concluded that ADHD could not be caused by lead exposure alone, and that lead is only one of the harmful chemicals to cause the symptoms of ADHD in humans. We can also say that a diagnosis of ADHD is not certain by increased lead exposure, but it can definitely be of some help in finding out the actual reason behind the symptoms.

Other Factors That Might Lead to ADHD

In this section, we are going to discuss various factors that might cause ADHD other than the ones already mentioned above.

- A study was conducted to find out whether ADHD can be caused by utero exposure to alcohol and smoking, and the research found that these are indeed risk factors of ADHD (Rosalind J. Neuman, 2007).

- Another study pointed out that preterm birth or babies who are born prior to their delivery date are also at risk of developing ADHD when they grow up (K. Lindstrom, 2011).

- There was a point of time when it was believed that symptoms of ADHD could be reduced if children were made to stop consuming food additives and refined sugar. And so, any food that contained preservatives, sugars, colorings, or artificial flavorings were not given to children. But NIH or National Institue of Research did a conference in the year 1982 where they declared that only five percent of ADHD kids were benefitted from eliminating sugar from the diet, and most of these kids either had food allergies or were quite young.

- In 2005, an article by Dr. Ruff was published in Clinical Pediatrics, where the term 'epidemic of modernity' was given to ADHD (Ruff, 2005). The article mainly focused on how the development of the brain in kids is affected by the type of life we lead today and the TV shows and video games that kids are exposed to. It was also mentioned that when kids are so into a fast-paced life on the outside, classroom teaching appears to be quite slow to them, and so, they start to treat their academic life with the same urgency that they display in the outside world.

Chapter 4: Diagnosis of ADHD

Have you not been able to finish any work this week? Do you keep losing your house keys all the time? Are you feeling terribly disorganized in your life? As you know, from Chapter 2, all of these symptoms definitely point to ADHD. But you also have to keep in mind that ADHD is much more than these symptoms alone. So, never jump to any conclusions before you visit a specialist. If you think about the different symptoms of ADHD singularly, you will realize that they are not really that abnormal. Feeling restless or forgetting things is very common. Even if your distractibility has reached chronic levels, it doesn't mean that you have ADHD.

The problematic part is that ADHD cannot be diagnosed through any physical or medical test. If you want to know whether you or your child is suffering from ADHD, you have to visit a specialist or a health professional who performs such a diagnosis. They implement a lot of different psychological tools to predict whether you have ADHD or not. They might ask you about your past problems or even the present ones, and you have to answer them honestly; they might even make a checklist of symptoms for you or prescribe some medical examinations that will help in ruling out certain other causes that might be behind those symptoms.

A proper diagnosis is very important because there are several symptoms like hyperactivity and loss of concentration that not only happen in ADHD but in a whole lot of other problems as well. This is why ADHD can be confused with a lot of other medical problems leading to a wrong diagnosis. It is also confused with certain emotional problems and learning disabilities just because there is an overlap in the symptoms. The problem with the wrong diagnosis is that the affected person will then not receive the treatment they deserve or require to cure their actual problem. So, keep in mind that just because your symptoms match with that of ADHD, it doesn't mean that it is ADHD. A thorough diagnosis aided with a properly researched assessment by a specialist is necessary to conclude it as ADHD.

Factors That Are Looked Into

Like I told you earlier, the specialist might you a set of questions that will help him/her to make a proper diagnosis. Every person displays different symptoms when it comes to ADHD. So, in order to make a proper diagnosis, there are different things that have to be considered by the professional and set the criteria accordingly. You should also promise yourself that you are going to be as honest as you can while answering the questions of the specialist; otherwise, the diagnosis will not be accurate.

In short, if someone has to be diagnosed with ADHD, they will have to show strong symptoms. These symptoms are a combination of inattention, impulsivity, and hyperactivity. They are known as the hallmark symptoms of ADHD. But just to give you an idea, some of the factors that the specialist takes note of are as follows –

- **What is the severity of the symptoms?** – If someone has to be diagnosed, then the symptoms that they are having should be severe enough to hamper their life to a great extent. It applies to both children and adults. If you see people who have already been diagnosed with ADHD, you will notice that multiple facets of their life have been gravely affected because of ADHD, and this includes their personal relationships, work, and even financial responsibilities.

- **Do the symptoms show themselves at a particular time?** – If you indeed have ADHD, then the symptoms will pop up in multiple settings and not just in one place. You will face symptoms at the workplace, at home, and even when you are out on a date. It is probably not ADHD if you are facing the symptoms at only one place or one time of the day.

- **When was the first time you noticed the symptoms?** – This is another very important thing to take note of in the diagnosis of ADHD. In the case of ADHD, the symptoms generally start appearing the childhood years. In some cases, people get diagnosed later on when they reach adulthood. Also, if you are an adult, then the therapist might help you trace your current symptoms back to the earlier years and help you think whether you faced them even before or not.

- **How long do you have the symptoms?** – This is somewhat related to the previous question, but here is something that you should know – if anyone is to be diagnosed with ADHD, the symptoms should be persisting for at least six months. It is only after that the specialist can rule it as ADHD.

How to Choose a Specialist for ADHD Diagnosis?

If someone has ADHD, whether it is an adult or a child, they are going to face problematic situations every day and so, getting them the right treatment is very important. There are a lot of specialists that you can go to for getting yourself or your kid diagnosed.

- **Primary Care Doctor** – The first option that is open in front of you is your primary care doctor or general practitioner. They will perform basic diagnosis, and depending upon the situation, they might either refer you to some psychiatrist/psychologist, or they can even prescribe medications.

- **Psychiatrist** – A psychiatrist is a highly trained medical professional in the scope of mental health. They are definitely one of the best people to help you with ADHD diagnosis and prescribe the right meds. They can even give you therapy and counseling sessions. If you are seeking a diagnosis for your child, then it is better that you visit a psychiatrist who already has experience working with kids in the past.

- **Psychologist** – When a health professional seeks a degree in psychology, they are referred to as a psychologist. They can offer you with different types of therapies like behavioral therapy and social skills therapy. They can even assist you in testing your child's IQ and, after that, take the necessary steps to mitigate the symptoms. In a few places, psychologists also have the power to prescribe medications, but in other places, psychologists are not always allowed to prescribe. In that case, they will ask you to visit a doctor who can prescribe meds.

Now, we come to the question – how are we to find a specialist who meets all our criteria and is right for us? This person should be someone you are comfortable with. Sometimes you might not find the right person at once. You will have to make appointments with some of them, visit them, and then decide for yourself whether you like them or not. That is why it is advised that you go to your primary care doctor, get an initial diagnosis, and also ask him/her for a reference. If you know someone who has ADHD, then you can also ask them for a reference. If it's your child who you think has ADHD, then you can also contact the school and ask them for a reference suitable for a child.

Your next step should be to call up your health insurance company. Sometimes these treatments are not covered, and at other times, they are. You can also ask them for names of specialists if the treatment is covered under the package. Once you have narrowed down to the prospective specialists, call them up, ask them for how long they have been practicing, and any other questions that you might have.

Here are some of the things that you can ask –

- What is their usual line of treatment for ADHD?

- Have they worked with children before, and if yes, then for how long?

- How can you make an appointment with the doctor?

Before you find the person who is a perfect fit for you, it is quite natural that you will have to do a bit of hit and trial. The person that you finally choose should be someone who has a welcoming attitude, and you think that you will be comfortable talking to them. If, after a few appointments, you or your child are still struggling with building a bond, then I think it is time that you look for another therapist.

Diagnostic Challenges

As already discussed, there are a lot of challenges related to ADHD diagnosis. The major one being that some people are not diagnosed in their childhood years. The symptoms are not expressed in the same manner in children and adults. The reason behind the complexity of the diagnosis process of ADHD is that it depends on a lot of historical data of the patient, and all this information needs to be accurate. The process of collecting all that data and ensuring that it is correct can be quite challenging and also a tedious task. AHD can develop anytime after the age of 12. And if the person who is going to the specialist is already an adult, then he is going have a lot of trouble remembering things that happened when he was 12 years old.

A multi-source assessment has to be made to make the results concrete. Thus, different sources have to be used. Some of the examples include – history of employment records from school, any interviews that the person might have attended, and so on. So, going through all the available records and looking for diagnostic clues everywhere is how a proper diagnosis is made. The developmental problems are going to become even more commonplace if the person has a family history of consistent ADHD. Any member of the family having ADHD completely changes the game because then the genetic factor is added.

Moreover, if someone does have ADHD, then they do not have the best memory, and thus, their accounts of what happened earlier cannot simply be trusted. When asked, they might say that they are facing problems in some aspect of their life when, in reality, nothing like that is happening there but in some other aspect of their life. So, do not trust anything that the patient has said unless and until you have cross-referenced it with something else. That is why diagnosis is advised to be done in a combination of feedback tests from colleagues, school records, and families.

The society that we live is provided us with a daily amount of stimulation that can lead to the formation of ADHD like symptoms. So, at any particular point in time, there is a lot of things on your plate competing to get your attention. On top of all that, you might also feel stressed because of your personal relationships. If someone lives in a dysfunctional family or works at a chaotic office, then it can not only cause inattention but also cause mood disorder.

The comorbidity rates in the case of ADHD are so high that it often causes a lot of confusion. It causes distraction, and people are no longer sure whether it is ADHD or not. There might be some obvious disorders in a person that is easily diagnosable, but he/she might also have ADHD that is subtle. In such a case, the diagnosis of ADHD is overlooked. Only a very patient diagnostician with an informed approach can rule it as ADHD if they keep an eye on all the other co-existing problems.

Another challenge that is faced is that certain drugs that are used in the treatment of ADHD have a tendency to induce addiction. So, there are people who tend to fake ADHD just because they want to get hold of those drugs. At the same time, this same problem might lead to a denied diagnosis of those who truly have ADHD. So, when someone is making a decision regarding the diagnosis of ADHD, they should be considering both sides of the story.

Here is something else that should be kept in mind – sometimes, patients are overpathologized by the diagnosis. That is not what an ideal situation should be. The ultimate aim of diagnosis is to give the necessary help to the person. The diagnosis should not convince the person that he/she is a failure, or it should not give them an excuse to give up on their lives. The diagnosis should be the first step towards selecting the most effective form of treatment for that person.

Step-By-Step Guide to Diagnosing ADHD

Here I am going to guide you through a step-by-step approach to ADHD diagnosis –

Social, Academic, and Emotional Functioning Assessment

This is the first step in ADHD diagnosis. The different aspects of life are evaluated, and this holds true for both adults and children. Once a detailed assessment report is made, it will be compared to kids who do not have ADHD to see what is abnormal and what is normal.

There will be checklists and questionnaires regarding the behavior of the patient – this is basically a self-report. In case the patient is a child, a 'report by other' is also done, and in that case, the questionnaires and checklists will have to be answered by someone who spends a lot of time with the child. Once all of these reports have been completed, a score is calculated. This score is the point of comparison to find out what is ordinary and what stands out and might be a possible symptom of ADHD. Several standardized rating scales are also used by specialists in order to evaluate the information. One of the most important parts of the comprehensive assessment of a child or adult is the behavioral checklist. But these reports cannot solely diagnose ADHD. They are just a part of the process.

After the behavioral checklists, it is time for the intelligence tests, which are also very crucial. There are some standard tests that are done first, and then once the findings arrive, some special tests might also be done depending on the findings. Tests of daily functioning, achievement tests, and intelligence tests are some of the common tests that are done. These can further include personality tests, memory tests, and symptoms checklists. There are two basic components of intelligence, and these are judged by these tests. These components are – the ability of a person to learn from what happened before and the ability to adapt to new situations. Basically, when these intelligence tests are conducted, the specialists are looking for any inconsistencies in the cognitive and behavioral patterns that are usually present in other disorders. One of the prime requirements of these tests is a consistent level of mental effort, which is something ADHD patients struggle with. The tests require a person to be fast-paced, attentive, and solid memory skills, all of which are not present in ADHD patients. Moreover, in most of these tests, the instructions are not repeated more than once. So, it is because of these tests that the intellectual functioning of a person can be judged.

Next, the achievement tests are usually designed to judge the person's skills in specific subjects. It can be mathematics or even oral language. Sometimes, diagnosing ADHD becomes easier because kids who have ADHD have a specific performance pattern in these tests. That pattern can then be used by experts to make a future diagnosis as well. Scores are usually high when a particular task does not require the person to engage in sustained effort. On the contrary, scores are low when the task requires sustained mental effort and concentration.

As you know that ADHD patients have trouble paying attention, and so, the next test done during the diagnosis are the tests of attention. Even though it might sound like an easy test for you, it is not. There are four different aspects of attention, namely, sustained attention, alternating attention, selective attention, and divided attention. In order to find what the weaknesses and strengths of a patient are, all the aspects of attention are tested.

Once this is done, we move on to the last test that is done in this step – the memory test. Although, apart from the memory test, some other small general tests are also done. The memory test examines not only the patient's long-term memory skills but also short-term memory. The tests measure their distractibility, delayed memory, retrieval from memory, and auditory and visual memory.

Clinical Interviews

The second step in the process of diagnosis is the round of clinical interviews. These interviews are constructed to get information about the patient's educational history, family, and other personal facts. Detailed histories are collected not only from the patient but also from the other close people in his/her life. Everyone might have a different perspective, and once this interview round is over, all the perspectives are arranged in order to form a complete picture.

Some of the information that is asked to the caregivers or parents of the patient are as follows –

- How have the symptoms been progressing ever since they showed themselves?

- When or under what circumstances did the symptoms first appear?

- Under what settings are the patients facing functional difficulties, and how severe are they?

- What impact are the symptoms having on the family and the patient?

- Is the family of the patient capable of giving him/her the care they need at this moment?

Once the initial interviews with the caregiver or the family members are over, the specialists will then talk with the patient. The patient will always have his/her questions about the situation. Listening to their side of the story is equally essential for diagnosis. It can be quite a challenging process, especially if the person is not open to the idea of seeking the help of mental health professionals. The age of the patient is a huge determining factor as far as the perspective is concerned. But this step is vital because it will make the patient more open to the idea of treatment, and they will gradually become comfortable with the process.

Medical History and Physical Exam

Now, no matter what diagnostic assessment we are talking about, it can never be complete without checking what the overall health of the person is. It is even more critical if the person has started showing the symptoms only recently. If the symptoms did not show themselves gradually and were rather sudden, then the cause might not be ADHD in the first place.

The medical history of the patient will be demanded as part of the routine process. So, if the patient has any pre-existing medical conditions like asthma, allergies, epilepsy, and so on, then they have to declare it. The specialist might also ask questions related to the presence of psychiatric illness in the family.

Once all of these processes are complete, the doctor will look through all the conclusive findings and determine whether the patient has ADHD or not.

Chapter 5: Treatments for ADHD

Both therapy and medication are used for the treatment of ADHD. Basically, a combination of both these things is what the patient truly needs to make the symptoms manageable. With time, the patient will realize that the symptoms are no longer so difficult to deal with in their day-to-day life.

What Are the Medications Used in ADHD?

In this section, we are going to talk about the major types of medications used in the treatment of ADHD. But I would like to remind you once again that these medications are in no way going to cure ADHD permanently because ADHD cannot be cured. Yes, you can alleviate the symptoms and make your life easier, but the condition will remain with you throughout life. Once you start taking the meds, you can readily divulge into new skills, be attentive, feel calmer, and also feel less impulsive. The dosage of medications also differs depending on the types of medicines that you have been prescribed. Some of them are meant to be taken daily, while others are supposed to be taken only when you have some important work.

Also, which medication is going to work for you is something that you will understand after a bit of trial and error. In the beginning, you might find that the medication is not working properly – that's probably because you are not taking the right medicines for yourself. The medicines are different for adults and children, and there are only a few drugs that are meant for both.

So, the different types of drugs that are used in the treatment of adult ADHD are mentioned below.

Stimulants

When it comes to the treatment of ADHD, one of the first things that doctors prescribe are stimulants, and the reason is that these drugs tend to show the best results on patients. In most cases, the initial dosage is low, and then after every week, the dosage is slowly increased. With time, you will reach a point where you try a perfect balance of therapy and meds and limit your overall side-effects and also learn how to keep your symptoms in check.

In the case of adults, the most commonly prescribed medications include Daytrana, Adderall XR, Focalin XR, Concerta, and Vyvanse, and all of these are categorized as long-acting stimulants. The effect of these medications last for at least ten to fourteen hours at a stretch, and so, they are enough to get a person through the day. Another benefit is that the patient does not have to remember taking too many pills or frequent pills. Moreover, with these meds, there is a gradual improvement in symptoms—it helps the patient merge in with their new lifestyle.

Once you have accustomed yourself to the medicine and your dosage has been fixed, going to the doctor from time to time for follow-ups is very necessary. It will help to keep a check on whether you have any side effects. It will also let you know whether the meds are working properly. After a while, your doctor might also put you off the meds for a while. It is to ensure that your body's reaction to it can be monitored. It will help the doctor understand whether you still need to continue the meds or not. The doctor might also suggest taking off from the meds periodically for short periods so that your body doesn't become fully dependent on them. If you don't do this, then the most common consequence is that you might need a higher dose.

Sometimes the symptoms seem to be going crazier, and that's when changing the time or dosage of meds is rewarding in most cases. Some of the most commonly seen side effects include panic, anxiety, jitteriness, dry mouth, sleeplessness, mood swings, and headache.

But you should also keep in mind that these stimulant medications are not suitable for everyone. In some cases, patients suffer from too many side effects to continue the meds. Also, you might be prescribed something other than stimulants if you have other conditions like psychosis, high blood pressure, anxiety, bipolar disorder, Tourette's syndrome, or problems related to substance abuse.

The most commonly asked question among patients and their families is whether the medications of ADHD can lead to substance abuse problems in people who do not have it. Well, the answer is no. When you follow the dosage prescribed by your doctor, you should be fine and not have any substance abuse problems. In fact, there is no proof that ADHD meds lead to substance abuse. It has been noticed that adults who undergo the treatment of ADHD are the ones who do not encounter any substance abuse problems as compared to the higher percentage of people giving in to substance abuse when they have an untreated ADHD.

Non-Stimulants

If the doctor decides that the patient should not be taking stimulants, then they prescribe non-stimulants. Sometimes, doctors give both stimulants and non-stimulants.

Non-stimulants are of three different types –

- **ADHD-Specific** – As you can understand from the term, these non-stimulants have been specially designed for ADHD, and the FDA has also approved them for ADHD.

- **Anti-depressants** – The next type of non-stimulants are the anti-depressants, which help in stabilizing some neurochemicals and alleviate the symptoms. These medicines are also prescribed to those who deal with both

ADHD and one of the following – mood disorders, anxiety, or depression.

- **Blood Pressure Medicines** – Yes, medicines used for regulation of blood pressure are also used in the treatment of ADHD because the ingredients of these medications are somewhat similar to those of non-stimulants.

So, let us talk about the non-stimulants that are ADHD-specific. One of the most common ones in this category is Atomoxetine, and it can be used for children, teenagers, and adults. This particular medication is mainly responsible for controlling the levels of norepinephrine and giving it a slight boost. The use of this medication helps the patient manage their hyperactive behavior and concentrate better. Two of the other medicines in this category that are approved for use in children are Guanfacine ER and Clonidine ER, and they can be administered to children between the age group of six to seventeen. They can be prescribed to adults as well. The use of these medicines helps improve memory, attention power, and impulse control.

There are certain advantages of using non-stimulants as compared to stimulants. Firstly, the non-stimulants won't lead to problems like loss of appetite, insomnia, or agitation. They are not addictive and won't cause substance abuse problems. Moreover, when compared to stimulants, these medications are much smoother, and their effect lasts for a more extended period.

But some people shouldn't be taking non-stimulants. I am going to break it down to you in detail below –

Atomoxetine is a drug that shouldn't be taken by people who –

- Have depression and take a particular drug called MAOI or monoamine oxidase inhibitor. Some common examples of this drug include tranylcypromine and phenelzine.

- Have been diagnosed with a specific eye condition known as narrow-angle glaucoma. This condition is quite dangerous because it can lead to complete blindness by putting unnatural pressure on the eyes.

- Suffer from liver or jaundice problems

- Are allergic to this medication or any of its ingredients in particular

Similarly, you shouldn't take the medicine Clonidine if you have faced some sort of allergic reaction after taking it.

On the other hand, Guanfacine shouldn't be taken by those who –

- Already consume other meds having guanfacine in it

- Are allergic to the medication or any of its components in particular.

So, here are some final thoughts on things you should keep in mind before taking non-stimulants. You need to inform your doctor if you have any of these conditions –

- You take any other medication for other health problems that require you to have sedatives, anti-depressants, antipsychotics, and blood pressure meds.

- You have an intense history of alcohol and drug abuse and dependency.

- You have shown symptoms of allergic reactions to any medicine in the past.

- You suffer from some medical problems related to blood pressure, kidney, jaundice, liver problems, mental health problems, seizures, glaucoma, and heart problems.

- You are planning to become pregnant, or you are nursing, or you are currently pregnant.

- You take any over-the-counter medication, herbal medication, or dietary supplements.

- You frequently have suicidal thoughts or get irritated too easily.

After discussing all the factors, if your doctor advises you that non-stimulants can indeed work for you, then you need to make sure that you take your medication daily as recommended by him/her. To find out whether the drug is working for you or not, your doctor might also prescribe some tests for you.

Now, let us see how or why blood pressure drugs can be helpful in case of treating ADHD. It is mainly because these medicines have been found to help with the symptoms of ADHD and also have fewer side effects. It has not yet been found as to how do the medications for high blood pressure help ADHD patients, but it is probably because of the soothing and calming effect they bring on some parts of the brain. But some commonly seen side effects of taking these medications include dizziness, headaches, low blood pressure, and drowsiness. But if you are taking these medications, make sure you don't miss the dose, and even if you do, you need to call your doctor immediately.

Lastly, we are going to see how anti-depressants work for ADHD patients. People who have both depression and ADHD are usually the ones taking these. They help keep the aggressiveness in check and also control hyperactivity. They have quite significant effects on improving attention. When these drugs are prescribed to children, it is noticed that they automatically become disciplined and take directions easily. But you have to keep in mind that when compared to stimulants, they don't work that well. The primary mechanism of the working of these drugs is that they increase the levels of certain neurochemicals in the brain. Some of these chemicals are dopamine, serotonin, and norepinephrine. But if someone has epilepsy or a history of seizures, then they can't take Bupropion. Also, anyone having a history of bipolar disorder is refrained from using anti-depressants.

Can Therapy Help?

ADHD can be treated with the help of therapy in children, adults, and teenagers. Moreover, if someone is facing problems like anxiety or panic attacks, then that can be addressed with therapy too. In this section, you will learn about the major types of therapies that are mostly used to treat ADHD.

Psychoeducation

This type of therapy can be helpful for people of all ages. The ultimate motive of psychoeducation is to simplify the idea of ADHD understandable to the patient. The patients are made aware of the different symptoms that they might face and also the effects of those symptoms on their day-to-day activities. This kind of therapy helps the patient to adjust to ADHD and cope with it while living a normal and well-balanced life.

Behavior Therapy

This therapy is mainly designed for children with ADHD. The therapy usually involves both parents and teachers as well. The children are introduced to the concept of rewards. Then that is used to monitor and control their behavior. So, parents are asked what kind of behavior do they want to teach their child? For example, some children might not be cleaning their room, so the goal of the therapy would be to teach the child to keep their room tidy. So, if the child follows through and does what he/she is asked to, then they will be given a reward in the end for their good behavior. It is how good behavior is encouraged in the child. When teachers are involved in this therapy, it is mainly about teaching the child different types of structural activities. No matter how little the progress is, you should always encourage your child and be positive so that their motivation stays intact.

There is another part of behavior therapy, which is called social skills training. ADHD kids often face problems dealing with social settings. So, situations are created during the sessions where the child has to do role-play and learn how they should react in that situation. The process is really fun, and the children get to learn a lot of important things.

CBT

CBT stands for Cognitive Behavioral Therapy, and this therapy can be very fruitful in adults as well. The therapist will walk you through the process, and you will learn to change your perspective of things. It, in turn, will help you improve your behavior in different situations. The therapist uses several strategies to change your thoughts about various incidents and how you react to them. CBT can be done in a group or individually.

Nowadays, CBT programs have become developed because they teach adults a lot of things – managing time, overcoming hurdles in executive functions, and also stress management. The behavioral skills that are imparted by CBT have been found to be more useful for the patients. In fact, research has pointed out that irrespective of whether the patient is under medication or not, CBT alone can do wonders for minimizing ADHD symptoms. Interpersonal self-regulation is another benefit of CBT, along with several aspects of self-management. All the irrational beliefs that the patient might have are challenged through CBT, and then with the help of proper discussions, those beliefs are negated.

So, these were the most common types of treatment options that are there for ADHD. But here is something that you should know – about 75% of the ADHD patients suffer from at least one other psychiatric problem during their lifetime. It can be substance use disorders, bipolar disorder, depressive disorder, anxiety disorder, or antisocial personality disorder. If the co-existing condition of the patient is severe, then the treatment for that is started first, and then ADHD is administered.

Remember that the goal of your treatment is not only to help you manage the symptoms but also to help you improve your overall quality of life.

Chapter 6: Living With ADHD

Almost every aspect of life is affected by ADHD. But there are some tips that you can follow in order to make living with the symptoms much more manageable. Everything around you might seem chaotic, but once you follow these tips, things will start falling into place.

ADHD in adults can make their lives seem overwhelming at all times. Whether it is the work deadlines that you have to complete or family gatherings that you cannot afford to miss, everything starts to seem like a burden. And dealing with this feeling day in and day out is hectic and stressful. There will be hurdles in every area of your life. It is going to lay a massive impact on your relationships, both personal and professional.

The quality of life is reduced to a great extent. But if you want to know about the specific aspects of your life that are affected by ADHD and how you can minimize the problems, keep reading.

Binge Eating

Binge eating or compulsive eating is one of the direct results of ADHD. It is mainly because the patients of ADHD struggle very much whenever they have to set some kind of discipline or limitation on their habits. And, eating is one such habit that tends to go out of control in ADHD. Moreover, in adults, the level of dopamine in the brain is also lowered when they have ADHD. Dopamine is responsible for giving your body the 'feel-good' feeling, and binge eating raises the level dopamine. So, automatically, it is quite natural for you to want to binge eat.

As you know, impulsivity is one of the main symptoms of ADHD, and this impulsivity applies to all spheres of the person's life, including eating. In fact, it has been found that compulsive eating or binge eating as a habit is five times more common in those who have ADHD. The cognitive functions of people with ADHD are very poor, and they cannot interpret the meaning of things like all of us. So, they cannot understand what other people are trying to tell them, and similarly, they cannot understand what their bodies are trying to say to them. Thus, when they feel bored or upset, they think that the feeling is because they are hungry. So, to combat that feeling, they reach out to food.

So, if you are facing the same issue in your life, then here are some ways in which you can combat it –

- An ADHD brain can be put to good use too, for example, to lose weight. When people have ADHD, it is not that their brain is not sharp; it just doesn't know when to stop. So, in order to lose weight, your focus should not be on eating less but on something more fruitful. You can place your focus on getting engaged in a new exercise schedule or making healthier meals daily.

- Now, let us talk about food temptations. ADHD patients are not good at showing resistance, and so you should avoid doing it altogether. Everyone has a particular type of food that they tend to overeat. Find out what is yours and then keep that specific food item out of your reach. Don't buy things that you know you might end up overeating. I am not telling you to altogether opt-out of eating ice-cream, but I am asking you to do so infrequently. If you keep ice-cream in the fridge, battling that temptation to grab the ice-cream tub, the first chance you get would be hard. So, if you really want to have ice-cream at some point, you can just go out and have some.

- Like I said before, people with ADHD often interpret boredom as hunger and overeat. So, you have to stimulate your brain and keep it engaged so that you don't feel bored. For this, you have to set a limit for a daily stimulation dose and make sure you meet the minimum limit every day. The more exciting tasks you do, the less you will be searching for amusement in food. I would like to remind you that watching television doesn't fall into this category of exciting tasks. Instead, TV can make you want to overeat, and it does not provide much brain stimulation as well.

- Don't forget to exercise. You don't have to perform any heavy exercise, but just a few moves that come naturally. It will give you an energy boost and also uplift your mood. Even if you are not feeling like it, make yourself get up and walk for ten minutes or so. By the end of those ten minutes, you will feel the tension leaving your body, you will have greater energy levels, and your subjective hunger will reduce too.

- The next thing that we are going to discuss is quite useful – schedule your eating times. When you have ADHD, your brain is often not aware of what you feel. The brain always tries to stay ahead of others, and this same tendency is what makes you feel disconnected from everything else. When you are too focused on something else, you don't have a sense of time, and you forget to eat. It, in turn, makes you more hungry, and you overeat. But setting reminders for eating can solve this problem. Make it a resolution to eat something after every three to four hours, even if it is a snack. This will stimulate your brain and will also relieve you from the restlessness.

- Even after you follow all these tips, you still have to teach yourself how you can stop eating. For this, fix a particular serving size and follow it. When you are eating, concentrate on how you feel and analyze each state of feeling that you are experiencing. This is called mindful eating, and this is going to help you a lot with respect to binge eating. Binge eating is mostly the result of the pleasure that we anticipate during eating. But when you eat, if you focus on truly enjoying the food rather than anticipating the next move and gulping down more and more, it helps. After every five minutes, check with yourself whether you like the food or not. Don't think about the next course of the meal but focus on what you are eating now.

- Lastly, even if you make a mistake and end up overeating once, don't beat yourself too much. If self-loathing and yelling at your own self would have solved everything, then you would have overcome compulsive eating long back. So, if you slip, just forget the past, learn from your mistakes, and start your healthy eating plan again.

Anxiety

Before we move on to how anxiety is caused because of ADHD, you need to understand that ADHD and anxiety are not the same. They are two different disorders. But how will you understand that you have anxiety apart from having symptoms of ADHD? Well, it's quite simple really – if you are into constant worrying that is ruining your day-to-day life and also preventing you from doing normal things, then you are suffering from anxiety. Some people even complain that having anxiety has made them feel that they are always on edge.

Remember that all of us feel anxious from time to time, but that doesn't classify it as an anxiety disorder. Having anxiety attacks is much more than that. It can make you feel frightened to unnatural levels; you will feel distressed and uneasy even when you are under normal circumstances. It has been found that among the adults who have ADHD, about 40-60% also have anxiety (Hechtman, 2008).

There are different patterns in which anxiety can show itself in ADHD patients – it can be in the form of behavioral changes, cognitive changes, mood swings, or any physical activity. When anxiety strikes, the symptoms are quite paralyzing, and resuming normal lie can become a real struggle. Whenever a person with ADHD thinks that there might be a negative outcome to a situation, they start avoiding things. Anxiety also hampers with proper decision-making skills and leads to procrastination. So, how can an ADHD patient deal with anxiety? Here's how –

- The first step is to find what your triggers are. Some people can pinpoint events that cause them to become anxious – it can be as simple as receiving phone calls to complex things like public speaking. Your path to managing your anxiety will become much easier once you identify the events that are triggering you.

- The next thing to ensure is that you are getting enough sleep. Anxiety is often triggered when the ADHD brain does not get proper rest. Make it a resolution to sleep for 7-8 hours at night. In case you cannot sleep after going to bed, you should consult your doctor. He/She might give you some medication that will help you sleep. You can also try meditation because that often helps in these situations. Another thing to try is to maintain a fixed time of waking up in the morning and going to sleep at night. But never make the mistake of taking meds without consulting your doctor.

- Follow a fixed schedule. Completing tasks on your to-do list is one of the biggest hurdles of ADHD patients, and when tasks remain incomplete, it causes anxiety. But this can be prevented if you make a schedule and abide by it. When you prepare this schedule, don't make it too tight. If the schedule becomes too hard to follow, then you will always be rushing to complete things and get anxious in the process. So, set goals that are realistic.

- Here too, I would like to remind you that exercising regularly can actually help you in reducing your anxiety. It has been proven in different studies (Elizabeth Anderson, 2013). Even if you have a busy schedule, make sure you do at least half an hour of some form of physical activity. If you haven't had an exercise routine in your life, then I would advise you to start small. Work your way up slowly, and then you can practice a couple of intense workouts if you feel like it.

- Journaling is a very effective way to relieve anxiety. It helps you take the stress off your mind. There are no rules when it comes to journaling – you can do it in whichever way you feel think is right for you. The whole idea of journaling is to be comfortable with your own thoughts and writing them down. You don't necessarily have to do it in a fancy way. But if you do like to take things up a notch and be artistic, then it is completely your choice. You can even note down all your thoughts that you want to discuss with your therapist on your next session.

- Lastly, have patience because treating anxiety is not an overnight thing. It takes consistent effort and weeks for you to figure out which line of treatment is working for you.

Substance Abuse

There are several instances where patients of ADHD have been found to have substance abuse problems. In fact, among the patients who are admitted to a treatment center for drug and alcohol abuse, 25% have ADHD. But why does substance abuse and ADHD go hand in hand? Well, for starters, most patients turn to substance abuse to get a hold on their life. ADHD brains have reduced amounts of dopamine, and using drugs or alcohol increases that level. Moreover, alcoholism and ADHD both are conditions that have the tendency to run in families. So, if an ADHD child has a parent who also had ADHD and alcohol abuse problems, then the child is very much susceptible to developing the same as well.

Once someone has developed substance abuse problems, the treatment process is extensive and difficult, so every effort has to be made to prevent the problem altogether. For this, you should start talking to the kids from a young age about avoiding illicit drugs and the dangers of substance abuse. For adults, if you want to set yourself free from the habit of self-medication, then you should exercise daily because it really helps. When you exercise, it helps in stimulating the ADHD and prevents you from getting bored. Your brain becomes more vulnerable when you are bored, so it is important to keep yourself engaged.

Sleep Problem

ADHD has been found to cause sleep problems in patients of every age. There was a study in 2006 that found out that children who have ADHD often show symptoms of daytime sleepiness, whereas children without ADHD don't (Samuele Cortese, 2006). There was another study that showed that sleeping disordered breathing was found in 50% of the kids diagnosed with ADHD (Natali Golan, 2004). There have also been studies that show periodic leg movement and restless leg syndrome, both of which disrupt sleep, are more prevalent in kids who have ADHD than those who don't (Avi Sadeh, 2006).

But the most common question that people have is that why does ADHD cause sleep problems? Well, there are a number of reasons behind this, and they are as follows –

- ADHD medication often consists of stimulants, and one of the side-effects of these medications is that they hamper the sleeping pattern. They tend t make you feel more energetic, and so you feel like you are awake at all times. Conditions become worse when you have chocolate, coffee, tea, or any other source of caffeine.

- Keeping a schedule is difficult for ADHD patients. They have a hard time dealing with distractions in their day to day life. Even when they go to bed, they have all these thoughts running in their head that makes it difficult for them to calm their brain. Since they cannot reach this relaxed state of mind, they find it difficult to fall asleep.

- ADHD patients also have other disorders at times like mood disorders, anxiety, and depression, and all of them add to the problem of not getting proper sleep.

The first thing that you should do is inform your doctor because sometimes, all you need is a change in your medications or your dosage, and you will be able to sleep well. Also, your sleeplessness might not be as simple as it means. It can be due to some other underlying reason, and only a doctor will be able to tell you that for sure. But if all other causes have been examined and ruled out, then you have to inculcate some healthy habits and manage your ADHD-related sleeping problem –

- Refrain from consuming any type of caffeine at least four hours before going to bed.

- Don't take a nap about four hours before you go to bed.

- Maintain a fixed time for going to bed every day.

- Start a bedtime routine that helps you to relax. The routine should not be too elaborate.

- If you cannot change your stimulant medication, then you should at least try to take these medications in the earlier part of the day.

- Make sure your bedroom is appropriately dark and quiet for you to have a good sleeping atmosphere.

- Don't spend too much time looking at screens before bedtime.

Stress

The symptoms of ADHD can easily trigger you to become stressed – it is quite common, and it happens with everyone. The list of things that can cause you to become stressed is endless. A constant state of stress is what many ADHD patients complain about. Slowing down in life is a big battle, and they cannot focus on important things. Additional stress is created when they constantly miss their deadlines or feel guilty about missing those deadlines. It also leads to an increased amount of frustration that keeps accumulating.

But there are ways in which you can reduce this stress and get a grip on your life –

- Stress is created when you keep blaming and guilt-tripping yourself every time you forget something or miss a deadline. Stop doing this right now. Remind yourself that you have ADHD, and it is in your neurobiology to forget things. If you are not seeking treatment for ADHD, then visit a specialist right away. You can even join an internet forum or local support group to talk and listen to other people who have ADHD. This will help you acknowledge the fact that you have ADHD. The more you do these things, the more you will see that you are not the only one in this world to be dealing with these problems. This realization, in turn, will reduce your stress.

- Practice physical activity. It can be anything – it can be a ten-minute brisk walk around the block or some free-hand exercises at home. When you do some physical activity, the brain releases a particular chemical known as serotonin. Serotonin functions opposite to cortisol (the hormone responsible for stress). Moreover, your body's threshold of withstanding stress also increases the more you exercise.

- The concept of time is seen as a fluid thing by most ADHD patients. Practice wearing a watch at all times or keep a table clock on your desk. You can even set the timer to go off after every hour to let you know that an hour has passed.

- You need to bring more structure into your life. Make it a habit to plan your day before going to bed. So, create a list of things that need to be done the next day and then prioritize them. You can also assign a particular time span to each of these tasks to make it more organized.

- Learn to say no and create healthy boundaries. Don't bite more than you can eat. Stress is often raised when you overbook yourself.

- No matter how busy your life is, learn to take breaks from time to time. Make it a resolution to go out with your friends every weekend at a dinner or a movie night. You can even plan your weekends around your hobbies or go for a drive towards the countryside.

By now, you must have learned that ADHD can make people stressed out and worry about petty things. It is not easy to lead a life with ADHD weighing down upon your shoulders. But if you follow these tips, your life will gradually become more manageable.

Chapter 7: How to Sharpen Your Memory When You Have ADHD?

People with ADHD often suffer from executive function (EF) deficits with some of the most profound impairments linked with working memory, fluid intelligence, processing speed, planning, vigilance, and response inhibition. These EF deficits can be seen as a sign of lower intelligence and can lead to reduced self-esteem, decreased professional or academic achievements, and reduced income. It is thought that the intelligence deficits seen in people who have ADHD are caused because of impairments in higher-order cognitive processes (like working memory) and not due to direct impairment of cognitive abilities.

A majority of people who have ADHD or ADD have problems with working memory. Occasionally most of us forget important dates or lose our keys or leave our wallet in the refrigerator. You might think that these happen because you are inattentiveness. However, when these turn into habits, you might have a poor working memory associated with ADHD. They might have problems with differentiating between important and unimportant cues, organizing, focusing, and recalling things. It might be hard for them to get started on tasks, and might become forgetful and get distracted easily. It is often impossible and frustrating for them to follow lengthy multiple-step directions. Sharpening your working memory can help strengthen a person's problem-solving skills, control impulsive behaviors, and improve their ability to focus.

What Is Working Memory?

The term "working memory" and "short-term memory" are often used interchangeably. You might have heard either of these terms before. The terms refer to a "temporary storage system" that is located in the brain to store various thoughts and facts while you are performing a task or solving a problem. It, thus, allows you to store information and thoughts temporarily in your mind so that you can use them whenever you need them to finish a task. Working memory helps you to hold facts and thoughts for long enough so that you can use it in a short while, remember what to do next, and concentrate on your task at hand.

You can consider working memory to be a shelf in your brain. For example, you have to go to the supermarket because you need bread, eggs, and milk. While you are shopping for these things in the supermarket, you suddenly remember that you have to buy cereal as well. So you go to the cereal aisle. However, having to buy eggs falls off your mental shelf as you focus on buying the cereal. You come back home with bread, milk, and cereal and realize that you have forgotten to buy the eggs.

The total number of things that you can accommodate on your mental shelf might be different than the number that another person can store in his working memory. Studies have revealed that young children can hold only one or two things in their working memory as they have limited working memory skills. It continues to develop until one reaches the age of fifteen. However, not everyone has the same capacity for working memory, and it doesn't develop at the same pace for everyone. Some people can accommodate more items in their mental shelf than others.

Scientists don't agree on the number of information "bytes" that the brain can hold. According to some, it's just around four, while others claim that it's as many as seven items. Several studies have also been conducted, which showed that one's working memory could be strengthened and improved. You can increase your capacity of working memory by grouping things together. For instance, a phone number generally consists of ten digits; however, we often divide the number into three separate groups. It helps us to remember the ten-digit number by making use of only three working memory slots. Working memory is similar to plastic – trainable, movable, and flexible. It is just like our muscles and can be improved with the help of training and exercise.

When Do We Use Working Memory?

Working memory is used by us in various situations every day. We use it to follow multi-step directions, do mental math, follow a conversation, organize, plan, write, or read. It helps us to stay engaged and focused on a task. Working memory is also important for students. Recent research conducted in the United Kingdom with around 3000 junior high and grade-school students revealed that struggles in school were caused mostly due to weak working memory and not because of low IQ. Studies also showed that almost all the students who had a poor working memory scored less in math and reading comprehension.

Here are some examples of how your daily life is affected by weak working memory:

- Your inability to follow through on projects and your disorganization causes you to miss deadlines at work.

- In order to retain information, you have to reread something multiple times.

- You plan to work from the comfort of your house; however, you don't remember to bring the items that you require with you.

- You get distracted and forget about the first project, and so have several unfinished projects.

- While having a conversation with someone, you forget what the other person has just said and so have difficulty following a conversation.

- Even when you were just told the directions to a place, you tend to get lost easily.

- You keep losing your wallet, cell phone, or keys.

- You wish to pitch in a conversation. However, you forget what you wanted to say by the time the other person has done speaking.

You require the help of your working memory no matter what you want to do.

You can use a number of services and products (for example, Play Attention and CogMed) to strengthen your working memory and train your brain. Several studies have revealed that such products and services can improve your working memory; however, the benefits might not last beyond the training session. Other studies have, however, shown that if you commit to training your brain, it can significantly improve your working memory.

The first step to strengthening your working memory is by understanding your own limitations and knowing how memory works. It does not mean you can excuse yourself by just saying that you are sorry. It means you can compensate for forgetting by developing and using certain strategies. People who have ADHD often try to keep things in order by using reminder systems. They might keep a list of things they need to buy at the grocery store or keep a running to-do list on a notepad app on their tablet or phone. They might also use a calendar app or a timer to remind them of their appointments.

Tips to Boost Working Memory

Here are some tips on how you can improve your working memory:

- **Include exercise in your daily routine** – According to a few studies, exercising regularly can improve your working memory. Researchers believe that physical activity and exercise can improve the health of brain cells. It can also reduce stress, help you sleep better, and improve your mood – all of which can indirectly influence your memory and affect your cognitive abilities.

- **Using mindfulness to strengthen your working memory and reduce distractions** – A research conducted by MIT, Massachusetts General Hospital, and Harvard Medical School found that exercising mindfulness techniques daily can improve recall and also allowed the participants to regulate their sensory output and tune out any distractions.

- **Decrease multitasking** – A research conducted at the University of Sussex found that multitasking can decrease particular regions of your brain and is also associated with a reduced attention span. Try finishing the task at hand before moving on to the next task.

- **Try different methods of remembering information** – Making up a rhyme or creating a song might make it easier for you to remember a list of things. Some might also find it easier to remember multiple things by visualizing them. Visualize yourself stopping at the grocery store when you are coming home from work and picking up yogurt, bread, cheese, and milk. Try to imagine what it would look like to go to each section of the store. You are more likely to remember all the items you need to purchase at the grocery store if you follow your visualization. It is because images and visuals can be more powerful than words.

- **Develop routines** – When you return from work, start by creating a routine. As soon as you walk through your door, choose a specific place to keep your keys and cell phone. Keep them in the same place every time when you return from work.

- **Use checklists for tasks that have several steps** – Try making a checklist for your first hour at work. It could include several tasks like reviewing yesterday's progress, checking and replying to emails, returning calls, listening to messages, checking with the supervisor for the necessary tasks that need to be finished immediately, etc.

- **Divide large chunks of information into smaller pieces** — Before moving forward to the next instruction, concentrate on one or two of them first. For instance, if you want to get ready to host a party in your house but are stressed and overwhelmed about everything that you need to get done like setting up for the party, cleaning the house, cooking, and shopping. Try concentrating on a single area at one time, like shopping. Forget about the remaining tasks until you have finished shopping.

- **Practice your skills of working memory** — You can create your own brain training programs or use the ones mentioned above. Note down six words that are unrelated to each other. Begin by trying to remember the 1st two words without seeing the paper. Then, as you succeed, add another word to the sequence.

Working memory is used by children all the time to learn things. They need it for things like solving math problems in their heads or following multi-step directions. You can help your kid strengthen their working memory by incorporating some simple strategies in their daily lives. Here are some tips by which you can boost your child's working memory:

- **Help make connections** – Help your kid create links that associate various details and make them memorable. Using fun mnemonics is another great way to grab your kid's attention. Finding ways to link different information also helps in creating and recover long-term memories. It can also help with working memory with which they can hold and compare recent and old memories.

- **Make it multisensory** – Processing information using multiple senses can help improve long-term memory as well as working memory. Note down certain tasks for your kid so that they can look at them. Let your child hear them when you say them out loud. Walk with your kid through your house while telling them about the family chores that they need to finish. When you use multisensory strategies, it helps your kids store the information in their minds for a long enough to use it.

- **Encourage active reading** – Highlighting or underlining text and jotting down notes can help children keep the facts in their minds for long enough so that they can answer questions about them. This is why sticky notes and highlighters are so famous nowadays. Asking questions about the text they are reading and reading it out loud can also help with their working memory. Long-term memories can also be formed with the help of these active reading strategies.

- **Play cards** – Easy card games like War, Go Fish, Uno, and Crazy Eights can help strengthen your kid's working memory in 2 ways. Not only do they have to remember and maintain the rules of the game they are playing, but they also need to keep in mind the cards they have and the ones the other players have played.

- **Play games that use visual memory** – Kids can improve their visual memory by playing matching games. You can also try giving your child a page from a magazine and tell them to mark all the instances of the letter "a" or the word "the." It can also be fun to use license plates and recite the numbers and letters on them and then taking turns to speak them backward as well.

- **Have your children teach you** – When you can explain how to perform or do something to others, it involves understanding the information and filling it mentally. For instance, if your kid is learning how to dribble a basketball, ask them to teach you how to do it. Teachers also do something similar to this when they pair up students in a class. Doing this allows them to begin working with the facts instantly instead of waiting to be called on.

Top Strategies for Improving Overall Memory

Everyone wants to have a better memory. Here are some simple strategies that you can use to improve your overall memory:

- **Cross lateral movements** – These kinds of movements involve using your legs and hands on opposite sides of your body. You can perform some of these cross-lateral movements for at least 5 minutes every day. This can help you improve your mental alertness and concentration power.

    o Double doodle: Try drawing a pattern or design using both your hands at the same time. Make sure that the designs are not facing the same direction and are mirror images of each other.

    o Cross crawl sit-ups: Lie on you back and keep your hands under your head for support. Then, sit up and touch your left elbow to your right knee. Alternate the movement by touching your right elbow to your left knee.

- Karate cross crawl: Use alternate hand and foot to kick while chopping or punching. For instance, when your left foot kicks, your right-hand chops.

- Lazy 8: Trace a large infinity sign in front of your body using one hand. Follow your hand with your eyes. Do it a couple of times and alternate hands.

- Try touching your elbow or hand to your opposite knee.

- **Movements help turn the brain on** – Finding fun and creative ways to include movement in your study time is one of the best ways by which you can stay focused and alert. Try doing any of the following movements given below for at least five minutes before starting your study or work sessions. Also, make sure to incorporate movement breaks into your sessions every fifteen to thirty minutes.

Try following low concentration, repetitive tasks like the ones given below.

- Squeezing a ball
- Rocking
- Folding a piece of paper
- Doodling

Try pulling, pushing, or stretching movements like:

- Pushing against the wall
- Stretching a big elastic band
- Tug of war

Balancing activates the same regions of the brain that also manage attention. Try spinning and balancing movements like:

- Standing on a balance board having rockers under it
- Walking around the room while studying or reading
- Turning around a couple of times in a particular direction and then altering the direction

Try joint compression movements like:

- Bouncing up and down in your chair
- Jumping jacks
- Jumping up and down

- **Capitalize on your natural processing skills** – Everyone has a natural style of processing information. Your superweapons are your natural approaches and your unique set of strengths. You can improve your memory by recognizing and making use of these skills and strengths. When you use your natural processing style, it helps stimulate your senses by making associations in your mind. If you are an auditory person, you can use rhymes, jingles, and songs, which will act as a framework to help you remember information. If you are a visual person, you might want to make vivid visuals in your mind. If you are a kinesthetic person, you can incorporate some movements into your mental image. If you think that you are affected by your tactile senses, you can put your sense of touch in your mental image. And, f you think you have a good olfactory sense, then you can incorporate different scents into your mental imagery.

These memory techniques work better when they are used together. You can build stronger associations in your mind by incorporating more of these sensory factors into your mental imagery. It can also increase the number of triggers you are leaving behind that can later help you in recalling the information. A multisensory approach can also help you in forming new memories. Try doing it every time you are studying. You can sing it, draw it, read it, write it, or say it. You can do whatever it takes to make it stick.

- **Analogies** – Creating new exciting connections to make the dry facts more personally relevant and meaningful to you is a great way to make things more interesting. For example, when you are trying to memorize the different cell organelles present in the body, consider a cell to be a city and link the function and name of each organelle to the characteristics of the city. For instance, the endoplasmic reticulum is the highway, the cytoplasm is the lawn, and the mitochondrion is the power plant. You can also make up a vivid story about a character in the city for added memory power. You can make the character interact with the other elements you have created. Creating a story will help cement the facts in your mind. Make sure to make the story a bit strange in some way so that it can grab the attention of your brain.

- **Mind mapping** – Creating mind maps that link different ideas helps you capitalize on the brain's ability to latch on to geometric shapes. A mind map makes it easier for many people to remember information. Making mind maps are very easy. Simply write your topic anywhere on a piece of paper and then brainstorm important ideas that you get and jot them down anywhere on the paper. Just link them to the ideas that they are connected to when they come to your mind.

Take some time each day to practice these strategies and then try to put them in your everyday life. You can experience an improvement in the effectiveness and efficiency of memorization by using these strategies.

Chapter 8: What Should You Know About the ADHD Diet?

Most people wonder whether they can improve their power to focus and treat the symptoms of ADHD by eating the right kind of food. Well, to some extent, yes, and that is what we are going to discuss in this chapter. Although there have been no conclusive studies in this field that say that nutritional deficiencies can lead to ADHD, the symptoms can definitely be managed by following a particular diet. There are certain food items that help and certain food items that you shouldn't eat.

What Is ADHD Diet?

Before going into too many details, let us see what the ADHD diet is all about. As you know, ADHD patients tend to become very energetic and hyperactive. This diet helps in alleviating those symptoms. Dr. Benjamin Feingold had suggested some changes to be made in the diet of his patients in the 1970s. These changes showed effectiveness in reducing symptoms of certain conditions like hives, asthma, and behavioral disorders. There have been several variations of the diet that Dr. Feingold created, and research has been done on all of them. There is no conclusive evidence on the reduction of ADHD symptoms. But there have been several patients who claimed that this diet really helped them manage their symptoms and lead a better life.

In Chapter 3, we studied the causes of ADHD in detail, and there, we saw that additives and colorings in food could increase the chances of developing ADHD. So, the ADHD diet encourages you to eliminate certain things from your diet like –

- Artificial flavorings. One of the most common examples is that of synthetic vanilla.

- Artificial colorings

- Preservatives. Some common examples are TBHQ or tert-Butylhydroquinone, BHT or butylated hydroxytoluene, and BHA or butylated hydroxyanisole.

- Salicylates or any other chemicals that are present in food naturally. Some food items include tomatoes, berries, and apricots.

- Artificial sweeteners. Some common names in this category are sucralose, saccharin, and aspartame.

Now, let us see some of the food items that have been strictly removed from this diet –

- Coffee
- Grapes

- Apricots
- Apples
- Almonds
- Mint flavoring
- Cloves
- Cherries
- Berries
- Prunes
- Plums
- Pickles and cucumbers
- Oranges
- Tomatoes
- Tea
- Currants
- Peppers
- Peaches
- Nectarines
- Tangerines

Here are some of the foods that you should eat on this diet –

- Beets
- Beans
- Celery
- Dates
- Bean Sprouts
- Lettuce
- Cauliflower
- Onion
- Mushrooms
- Pears
- Honeydew
- Sweet potato
- Grapefruit
- Carrots
- Cantaloupe
- Mangoes

- Kiwi
- Kale
- Squash
- Potatoes
- Pineapple
- Peas
- Zucchini
- Watermelon
- Spinach
- Bananas
- Cabbage
- Brussels sprouts
- Lentils
- Lemons
- Sweet corn

Once you practice these eating habits, you will notice a marked difference in your symptoms of inattentiveness and restlessness. Some of the choices that you have under this diet are as follows –

- **Elimination Diets** – When you follow this type of diet, you are consciously choosing not to eat those foods which have been proven to trigger the ADHD symptoms. A list of such food items has already been mentioned above.

- **Supplementation Diets** – In this plan, the goal is to supplement your foods with a variety of nutrients, including vitamins and minerals. When you take these supplements, any deficiency that might have formed in your body will be overcome. This plan is supported by those who strongly believe that a shortage of certain nutrients in the body can trigger the symptoms of ADHD.

- **Overall Nutrition** – This plan is based on the assumption of both of the plans mentioned above. You will be eating some foods that are responsible for making you feel good and relieve you from your symptoms, and you will also be eliminating certain food items that are harmful to your symptoms.

Even though the data is relatively limited with respect to the ADHD diet, there are certain things that experts believe after extensive research. They think that following these tips might help the patients get relief from the symptoms. The main thought behind this is that whatever food item boosts brain health is also good for combating ADHD. So, you should eat –

- *A diet rich in protein* – There are so many good sources of protein that you should consume. It includes cheese, beans, nuts, and even meat. Protein should be included in your breakfast to give you a healthy and energy-boosting start, and it should also be included in your snacks. There is a possibility that protein-rich foods help in extending the effect of the ADHD medications on your body. They also help in increasing your level of concentration.

- *Complex carbohydrates* – These are one of the healthiest things and should definitely be included in your diet. For this, you have to include fruits and vegetables like kiwi, apples, tangerines, tomatoes, and so on. The complex carbohydrates should be preferably consumed in the latter part of the day, or in dinner because they boost your sleep.

- *Omega-3-fatty acids* – These are another group fo very healthy nutrients that no one should miss. You will find them in fishes like salmon, tuna, and whitefish. They are also present in canola oil, olive oil, brazil nuts, and walnuts. If you think that your diet is not being able to provide you with a sufficient amount of omega-3-fatty acid, then you should consider taking a supplement. As a part of the ADHD management plan, Vayarin is an omega compound that is widely used, and the FDA has also approved it.

Sample Meal Plan

If you are not sure as to where you can start, then here is a sample meal plan that will save your time and also give you a boost of energy for the day –

- **Breakfast** – Whole-wheat toast with some eggs and avocado; some coffee or tea, preferably herbal tea

- **Snack** – Chia seed pudding or fat-free yogurt with berries or fruits of your choice

- **Lunch** – Quinoa with baked chicken or salmon along with a salad of bell peppers, cucumbers, mixed leaves, and toppings can be of your choice but make sure you sprinkle some sunflower seeds on top

- **Snack** – Peanut butter and apple or apple and cinnamon

- **Dinner** – Brown rice with a curry (vegetable or chicken)

- **Dessert** – If you want dessert, then you can have an ounce of dark chocolate, or you can have a warm cuppa of herbal tea before sleeping.

Best Foods for the ADHD Diet

I had given you a rough list of foods that you can eat on this diet, but here, we are going to see the different food items categorized into different nutritional groups. We are also going to see how these particular group of foods help in managing the ADHD symptoms.

Protein & Complex Carbs

ADHD symptoms are relieved to a great extent when you include more protein in your diet. As you might already know, the brain releases certain chemicals in your body, which are known as neurotransmitters, and these chemicals are the ones that are responsible for carrying the messages from one part of the brain to another. Now, for the body to produce neurotransmitters, protein is required. Apart from this, the symptoms of impulsivity and hyperactivity are often linked with a rise in the level of sugar in the blood. It can be prevented by increasing protein intake. In fact, this is also why it is advised that your breakfast should be rich in protein. But that's not all. Try different ways in which you can insert some protein in your diet throughout the day. You can have berry smoothies or protein bars, which are not only tasty but also great options for protein intake throughout the day.

Complex carbs, on the other hand, help in reducing the chances of a spike in blood sugar. When you consume more complex carbs, your satiety levels are increased, and you stay full for longer hours. It means your urge to grab on those sugar stuff whenever you feel hungry will reduce. Moreover, consuming complex carbs before going to bed has shown proven effects on better sleep.

So, here are the food items that you should include in your diet to enhance protein intake –

- Lentils and beans
- Poultry and meat products
- Shellfish
- Fish
- Nuts
- Eggs

Some of the examples of complex carbohydrates that should be included in your diet are as follows –

- Lentils and beans
- Brown rice
- Pasta and whole-grain bread
- Vegetables
- Fruits

Vitamins & Minerals

Vitamins and minerals are very important for your body, irrespective of whether you have ADHD or not. They help in improving your alertness and also improves attention.

There have been studies that show ADHD is also linked with deficiencies of certain vitamins and minerals (Amelia Villagomez, 2014). But there is no conclusive evidence stating that a deficiency of any minerals or vitamins leads to ADHD. However, it is also true that when people increased their consumption of these vitamins and minerals, they witnessed a positive change in their symptoms. So, to be on the safe side, there is no harm in increasing your consumption of these nutrients.

Here is a list of food items in which you can find the specific nutrients –

- **Magnesium** – Almonds, pumpkin seeds, peanuts, and spinach
- **Zinc** – Nuts, beans, meat, and shellfish
- **Iron** – Tofu, kidney beans, beef, and liver
- **Vitamin D** – Fortified foods, beef liver, egg yolks, and fatty fish
- **Vitamin B-6** – Potatoes, peanuts, fish, and eggs

The regulation of dopamine in your brain is controlled b zinc. In fact, zinc might even be responsible for producing methylphenidate. This particular compound is, in turn, responsible for improving the response of the brain towards dopamine. Inattentiveness has been found in patients who had lower levels of this mineral. Similarly, iron is yet another mineral that holds importance in the production of dopamine.

Iron stores in the body are measured through a compound known as ferritin. A study was conducted, and it showed that ferritin levels were in 18% of kids in the control group as compared to the 84% of kids with ADHD (Eric Konofal, 2004). The symptoms of ADHD have been found to become severe when iron stores were low. The cognitive defects increased too.

Magnesium is responsible for inducing a calming effect, and it is also involved in the production of certain neurotransmitters. Thus, the intake of magnesium helps in increasing concentration and attention.

Omega-3-Fatty Acids

These compounds are very important for promoting healthy nerve function and also for keeping your brain in good health. A study was conducted in Sweden, and it found that ADHD symptoms were decreased by 50% when omega-3s were consumed daily in the form of fatty, cold-water fish like salmon, tuna, and sardines (Mats Johnson, 2009).

Dr. Sven Ostlund selected a group of children, and these children were in the age group of 8-18. They consumed fish oil every day. A 25% reduction of ADHD symptoms was noticed in these children within a span of 6 months.

There was another study that showed – the process of breakdown of omega-3s is much easier and faster in patients with ADHD than in those who are not diagnosed with this disorder (Genevieve Young, 2005). Greater levels of improvement in terms of cognitive function and mental focus were observed in those ADHD patients whose levels of omega-3s in blood were low. But you also have to remember that consuming omega-3s doesn't mean they can substitute your normal medications.

Some of the common food items that can provide you with omega-3-fatty acids are as follows –

- Flax seeds
- Chia seeds
- Walnuts
- Tuna and salmon and other fatty fish

If you think that food alone cannot provide your body with the required amount of nutrients, then you can also try taking daily supplements. Talk to your doctor about which supplement will be good for you.

Chapter 9: Tips to Make Your Life More Organized

One of the biggest challenges when a person has ADHD, is to become organized. But it is not something impossible. You can bring structure and discipline to your life if you put in the effort. Always remember that the secret to becoming organized is to follow some simple steps that you can continue doing and having a system that works well for your routine. In this chapter, we are going to have a lot at some simple tips that will help you make your life more organized.

Throw Out What You Don't Need

We all have things in our lives that we keep on accumulating even though we don't need them. And in the case of people with ADHD, these things are even more because they have very poor organizational skills. The more physical clutter you have in your life, the more will be your mental clutter. So, it would be best if you eliminated all those things you don't need from time to time. If you can't figure out where to start, then here are some things that you can throw away –

- **Plastic Grocery Bags** – These things tend to get accumulated in our houses very easily. If you are feeling like going green, just take all the plastic bags that are lying around and visit the nearest recycling center. Then, visit the supermarket and buy some reusable grocery bags. Keep about five of them in your car so that whenever you go somewhere, you always have one in the car. You should buy a bunch more to keep in your house. But in case you are at a store, and you don't have your reusable bags with you, you can always ask for paper bags.

- **Extension Cords** – I know that most of us are guilty of keeping worn out extension cords in our home. But ask yourself whether you really need so many of them. You can just keep one from each type of cord and throw away the rest.

- **Old Electronics** – Do you hold on to your old gadget even when you have bought a new one? That is how you are giving rise to clutter. You need to get rid of the old one. Or, you can also replace your old one and get a new gadget – this might even save you some money.

- **Extra Bedsheets** – Open your linen closet and see how many bedsheets you have. Every one of us keeps extra bedsheets in case we need them when guests are over. But do you have too many? If so, then you need to discard some of them.

- **Manuals** – In today's when you have everything you need online, why keep accumulating manuals? The first page of the manual might have the warranty card – you can tear it off and throw the rest of the manual away. Even if you need to know something about your device, all you need is the model number, and you will find every information online.

- **Free Samples** – Do you feel good when you get free samples with other products or when you travel? Of course, you do but think about all those times when these free samples just keep accumulating, and we never really use them. So, instead of throwing these samples away, you can donate them to those who really need them.

- **Magazines** – Do you have magazines lying around in every room? If yes, then you need to make a list of magazines that you really love to read, and anything that is not on that list should be recycled. Also, prioritize the magazines to see whether you still want to continue your subscription to all of them.

Set a fixed day every month when you will go through your belongings and throw out things you don't need. After that, your focus should be on buying things that you absolutely need. If you don't buy unnecessary things, you will not have clutter in the first place.

Maintain a Planner

When you have ADHD, you often tend to forget things, and that creates even more chaos in life. But a simple solution to this problem is maintaining a planner. So, if you have been feeling that there is not enough time in the day for you to do everything, a planner can sort that out for you. You can now keep every errand, every meeting, and every event scheduled so that you don't forget about it. Make sure you keep some time extra on your hands when you note down the event in your calendar. If the meeting is at 2 pm, note down the time as 1:45 pm, so that you have some extra time to give you a cushion.

Once you start maintaining a planner, you will see how your personal and professional life undergoes a huge change. You are going to become so much more productive and no more putting off things for later. If it is included in your planner, you have to do it now. Whatever task we are talking about, a planner will help you stay ahead of things and keep some extra time for you and your family at the end of the day.

Constantly feeling overwhelmed is something very common with ADHD patients, and this leads to an immense amount of stress. But your schedule can be so much less hectic if only you maintain a planner. Every responsibility will be completed seamlessly. You can also use your planner to keep track of what you are eating and whether or not you are doing some regular exercise.

Another important thing to keep in mind is that even when you are maintaining your planner, you need to keep checking it from time to time to ensure that you are not missing out on anything. Make it a habit to note down all your meetings and appointments in the planner. If you don't want to do it manually, you can also use an app for it. Then, you can set timely reminders for everything that is on your planner.

Organize Your Finances

The next step to becoming organized is to have a look at your finances and make sure everything is in order. The forgetfulness that comes with ADHD often makes people overlook their finances, and by the time they realize that it needs work, it is too late. If you don't want that to happen to you, I think you should review your finances every quarter. Mark a particular date in your planner or calendar when you want to review all your financial statements and make sure you do those things on that date. This should be a comprehensive review and must include your retirement accounts, all your bank accounts, and your investment accounts.

If you do not use online banking, then it is high time that you do so now. It is going to make your life so much easier. Writing checks and doing all the work manually is such a hassle. But when you do it online, it becomes way easier. If you think about all the monthly bills that you have to pay, then online banking can make it a cakewalk because they can be paid automatically. If you are not so savvy with computers and that is what is pushing you back from online banking, don't worry, it's not that tough. But in any case, you can always ask a family member or a friend for help.

Sort through your credit cards and see what you need and what you don't. The more cards you have, the more you will get confused. So, it is always better to stick only a few cards that will give you more benefits than the others. If companies are bothering you with new card offers, read the terms very carefully and then judge whether you truly need them or your current card is enough to cover everything.

Always have a few hundred dollars in your apartment in someplace safe. This will serve as a backup in case the ATMs are closed, or there is a power outrage. If you keep misplacing your wallet every day before leaving the house, try using a wallet that is colorful. When your wallet is black or brown in color, they tend to mix with other things, and you cannot spot them at once. But when it has a bright color, it becomes easier to spot them.

Prioritize Your Happiness and Health

Most people don't realize how important it is to put their health before everything else. No matter where you are, you should always have some extra ADHD medication at hand. Whenever you are writing things in your planner, make sure you check your medication and note down the date when you need to refill it. In this way, you will never run out of medication. You can even set a reminder alert on your phone to remind you when you need to buy new meds. But the date you are setting for refilling your medication should be at least a week before you run out of meds.

Your schedule should not only be about work. You should keep ample space in your schedule for socializing. Taking care of yourself also means that you need to meet people and go out with them. If you are an avid reader, then join a book club. If you love fitness, join a yoga class. Do what you love but make time for yourself.

Another thing that really helps ADHD patients is joining ADHD support groups. These groups can do wonders to how you see your life. They provide a lot of emotional support on days when you don't feel like doing anything. Everything that you are going through, the group members have gone through as well. So, why not share your experiences? There are a lot of in-person and online groups that you can check out.

Make Decisions Within a Time Limit

Making decisions can be quite overwhelming for an ADHD patient, and the main reason behind this is that they end up being so confused that making a decision seems next to impossible. Some patients can even spend weeks agonizing over the same issue over and over again. However, when analyzed by someone else, those decisions should not take you more than a couple of minutes. If you are going through the same thing, then one of the simplest was to solve it is to set a time limit. When you have a time cap, you know that you have to make a decision by the end of that time cap. If you are deciding on which sofa you should buy, set a time cap and then make a resolution that you are going to make your final decision before your time cap is over.

Whenever you are making a decision, I know that there are a lot of factors and, thus, a lot of angles to think from. But you need not think about everything. You have to prioritize and think about only some of the factors which are most important to you. It can be practicality, price, aesthetics, or anything else. The factors should be chosen by their importance. Stick to one factor for your ultimate decision.

Don't Over-Commit

We all have a tendency to overcommit. But you have to hold yourself back from doing so. When people have ADHD, they have a hard time keeping track of everything in their life. So, when you over-commit, you have a lot of things on your plate, and you cannot possibly handle all of them. If you spread yourself too thin, none of the tasks can be completed properly. So, commit to one task at a time and don't take up too much work at a time. You have to prioritize your own mental health over anything else.

Your To-Do Lists Should Not Be Too Long

Making to-do lists is definitely a great way to start the day and keep track of all those things you need to do, but it is also very easy to get lost in them. So, it is my advice to you that you keep your to-do lists short. Your list should have the tasks written in bold and big letters and don't list more than five or six tasks on the list. If there any additional tasks, write them on the back of the index card, and you will do those tasks only if you have time left after completing the major ones. When you see that your list is becoming short and you don't have too many things on the same page, you will automatically feel less frustrated. This will make completing tasks much easier.

Limit Your Distractions

There are too many distractions in our everyday life, but there is a way to fight them. You simply have to take the first step. Organizing your life will become way too difficult if you don't steer clear of all the distractions. When you are working, your focus should be solely on your work. Put your phone in the silent mode, and don't look at it for the next fifteen minutes. You can check your email after that and then return back to work for another fifteen minutes. Free your workspace of any clutter. The more things you have on your desk, the more will be the distractions.

Lastly, I would say that you need to take it one project at a time. Once you have set your priority, focus on completing that before moving on to something else. This will ensure that before you start a new task, all the loose ends have been tied up. If you follow all these steps, you will gradually see that you are mastering the art of organization.

Chapter 10: ADHD Anger Management Tips

There are quite a handful of reasons why people with ADHD struggle to keep their anger in check. If you are struggling with it as well, then you will find a lot of strategies in this chapter that will help you overcome it in no time. One of the major reasons why anger is such a big issue in ADHD patients is the constant mood swings. At one moment, the person is happy and cheerful, and the next moment, they are feeling unsettles and furious. This makes them act in an impulsive manner. Another reason for such anger outbursts is the accumulation of stress in ADHD patients.

Remember that you are not the only one struggling to bring your anger under control. There are plenty of other people like you who are also trying to keep their anger in check. So, here are some constructive ways in which you can manage your anger.

Know What Makes You Angry

So, the first step to overcoming anger is to understand what is making you angry. In simpler terms, you have to identify your triggers. Anger can be triggered in a variety of situations, and it is not always the same for everyone. When you know the situation in which there is a chance of you getting angry, you can take a break and calm yourself down.

Whenever you figure out that something is triggering you, note it down. Since ADHD patients have very low impulse control, triggers can take a completely different form and pose far greater challenges. Some triggers are huge, while some are small and minute things.

Once you have made a list of your triggers, it is time you sit down and sort through them one by one. For each one of them, think as to how you can avoid the triggers, and in case you come face to face with it, think of strategies that will help you to keep your anger in control. For example, if you get triggered every time you are stuck in traffic, then you need to change your commute time. For this, you can talk to your employer. But always have a backup plan for every trigger in case the first plan doesn't work.

In case nothing works, you should call up someone you trust or rely on. Let them know beforehand that you are going to call them. Ask that friend to take your mind off the issue that is causing the anger. But if you can't get hold of anyone at that moment, try counting from one to ten slowly and take deep breaths.

Take Care of Yourself

You must be wondering how this is related to managing anger. Well, it is because anger doesn't come to you overnight. It results from keeping things inside of you for too long. It happens because you are not taking care of yourself or not noticing the things you should on a daily basis. This means that you need to sleep well. A good sleeping regimen can do wonders for your mood and also increase your threshold for anger. You also need to eat the right kinds of food. A healthy diet is so essential. Also, if you are on any medication for ADHD or anything else, make sure you don't miss out on them.

When you are taking care of yourself, you are giving your body everything it needs to stay well. Your body can function properly only when it gets what it needs. All of these small steps, when seen together, can reduce your symptoms and also help keep your anger in check.

Take Breaks

The next step for anger management is taking breaks. No matter how many things you have on your to-do list, you have to take breaks in between. You will easily burn out if you don't relax and take some rest. Work is important, but so is rest. If you keep the engine of your running for a long time, it is going to wear out soon. The same thing applies to your body. If you want to function healthily, you have to take breaks in between. This will give your mind time to reenergize and feel better. You need to give your spirit the time to refuel so that your anger outbursts don't happen at the most unfortunate moments. What may seem like a subtle grievance now might keep accumulating and take the shape of a serious anger outburst later.

Breaks should not be a once in a while things. They should be incorporated into your routine in a regular manner so that you don't forget about them. You need to take a break after every hour of work, after every week, after every month, and also after every year. The duration of each of these breaks will be different. You need to plan something special for yourself once a month and a grand trip once a year. It will help you freshen up your mind and return to work with more energy.

Think About the Consequences

This strategy has seemed to work for a lot of people. One of the most common things that you will notice in people with ADHD is that they are not able to control their anger outbursts. In simpler terms, they do not have restraint. That is why you need to take a pause and then think about what your anger is going to bring you. Is it good? The most probable answer is no. Then, take a moment to think about what is you acted in a better way? What if you changed your response to something positive? You should also try to talk to your coach or your friends and discuss the incident that triggered your anger. It might even lead to some self-revelation. You never know what helps in your growth so that the next time it happens, you can respond in a better way.

But if you are indeed in an unbearable situation, then you need to take a step back and think about the worst outcome. Well, the worst result might not even occur, but you should always be ready with a plan in case it does. Moreover, like you already know, regulation of emotions is something ADHD patients face a lot of trouble with. So, this exercise can be beneficial to them.

Always Remain Positive

We are now going to discuss an essential step. Staying positive is crucial to deal with all problems in your life. You are bound to come across situations in your life where people will push the buttons, and your anger will cross the threshold. But how you choose to act in that situation is what is most important. When faced with failures, ADHD patients end up overreacting most of the time. That is why having a plan for every situation is important. You also need to have a Plan B in case Plan A does not work. It will make sure that you do not dwell on your failures and always have a path that will help you move on.

One of the key steps to being positive is to pat yourself on the back and congratulate yourself from time to time. Every time you are successful at reigning in your anger and taking control of the situation, congratulate yourself. You deserve that. Your self-esteem will benefit a lot from this exercise, and gradually, you will notice that your relationship with others is also improving.

Learn to Express Yourself in Other Ways

There are a lot of ways to let your anger out than yelling, shouting, or creating a scene. For this, you have to acknowledge that anger is nothing but an emotion, and it is sending a signal to you that something is really bothering you. When you do that, you will be able to articulate yourself in a better way and, thus, express yourself without hurting someone. It would help if you simply made others hear you, and for that, an angry outburst is not a solution. You need to able to have a proper conversation. For this, you can learn to use the right words. An anger outburst is ingrained in us from a young age because when we are young, anger is how we express our feelings for which we don't have words. But when we grow up, we do have the words, and yet we turn to anger. You have to replace anger as your coping mechanism with something that won't hurt others and also take your pain away.

If you are too angry to talk to someone, then it is better that you don't talk to them at that moment. Reschedule your meeting and speak with them some other time when you are not angry. It will help you analyze their point of view without jumping to any conclusion.

At the beginning of this chapter, I told you that you need to know about your triggers. Similarly, you also need to learn about what calms you down. Everyone has a different strategy that works for them, and you need to find yours. If listening to music calms you down, then be it. If a walk around the block to take in the fresh air is what you need, do it. It is like your anger first aid kit, and you need to know your tools.

But to get started with anger management, you need to acknowledge to yourself that you are having a hard time controlling your anger. If nothing works, you should talk to your doctor about it.

Conclusion

Thank you for reading *Thriving With ADHD Workbook: Guide to Stop Losing Focus, Impulse Control and Disorganization Through a Mind Process for a New Life.* I sincerely hope that this book was able to give you the tools you were looking for, and you were able to clarify your doubts.

Now you have to take your baby steps towards working out all the problems you are facing at living your life with ADHD. So far, we have covered the major aspects of everyone's life and the most common problems that ADHD patients deal with. I want to close with a simple note that sometimes, along your journey, there will come the point when you need to seek help from others. And there is no need to shy away from that. We all need to seek help once in a while, and that is completely okay. That doesn't make you small or inferior. It only makes you stronger.

The symptoms of ADHD can easily overwhelm you and weight you down. If you don't deal with them, they will keep haunting you and hampering your life. By now, you must have understood that the functioning of an ADHD brain is quite different from others. There are different processes that lead to different behaviors. The great impact of these symptoms on a person's emotions is what poses as the major struggle.

It is time that you stop beating yourself up and start taking action towards leading a better life. I know that you must have heard comments like 'loser' and 'incompetent' from your colleagues or friends. But you cannot let these petty comments define you. Stop the negative thinking right now and replace it with positivity. I know that there are a lot of obstacles in your path, but you have to learn to deal with them one by one. If you try to handle them all at once, you will become overwhelmed. At the same time, you need to take your medication on time because the medications, together with therapy, is what will give you dramatic improvement.

Don't judge yourself too harshly – it is never healthy. The emotional pain can get too much, but you simply have to find ways to deal with it. I hope the strategies mentioned in this book help you get through some of the toughest moments. It is easy to beat yourself up, but it is not easy to forgive and move on. With ADHD, it is natural for you to feel self-critical at all times. The root of this problem lies in childhood because that's when ADHD kids are looked upon with displeasure from their teachers and parents. ADHD kids work day and night to get the approval of others, but it is never enough. But now that you are an adult, you need to break free of that cycle, and the strategies mentioned in this book are going to help you a lot.

Stop spending time thinking about your weaknesses because now, you need to focus on your strengths. Make yourself feel good. Take a notepad and make a list of all those things that you are good at. This will not only help you uncover your strengths but also show you that you are good at so many things.

People with ADHD have a hard time saying no. Even after you have followed all the strategies mentioned in this book, you will struggle if you cannot set boundaries. Don't let the people in your life walk all over you. There has to be a line that you cannot let others cross. Spend time with people who support you and who have the same qualities as you. This will make the process easier. When you are hanging out with people who see the best in you and support you the way you are, you will automatically feel happier.

Having said all this, I would like to remind you that you should take time off every week for yourself. During this time, do all the things that you love to do. This can mean anything – going on a road trip with friends, a backyard barbeque party, or even going to a book club. It is very similar to recharging batteries.

You cannot run away from the fact that your mood is going to change after every few minutes. But you need to come up with better ways to deal with those changes. Don't put the blame on someone else or waste time thinking about why you have mood swings. You need to figure out what you can do to tolerate that moment and spend it doing something that doesn't involve hurting others. You can go and play tennis or have a coffee at your favorite café.

The ADHD brain is wired to dive deep into the all-or-nothing thinking process. Giving structure to your life helps with ADHD symptoms, and I have included plenty of ways in this book in which you can do. Understand that your brain is biologically different from that of others and so you react differently to situations. After a certain point of time, ADHD patients get accustomed to the constant criticism hurled at them. But it would help if you stood up for yourself because you have done nothing wrong. And while you do that, celebrate all the small victories down the road. Every little success counts because you are putting in a lot of effort, and you deserve to be appreciated. I want to end this book by saying that you should find your own tribe and connect with more people who have ADHD through the various support groups. Connecting with others who have the same problem will not only make you feel understood but also appreciated.

Finally, I would be grateful if you left a review on Amazon if this book was able to provide you with the information you were looking for!

References

Ajay Singh, C. J. (2015). Overview of attention deficit hyperactivity disorder in young children. *Health Psychology Research, 3*(2).

Amelia Villagomez, U. R. (2014). Iron, Magnesium, Vitamin D, and Zinc Deficiencies in Children Presenting with Symptoms of Attention-Deficit/Hyperactivity Disorder. *Children, 1*(3), 261-279.

Avi Sadeh, L. P.-H. (2006). Sleep in children with attention-deficit hyperactivity disorder: a meta-analysis of polysomnographic studies. *Sleep medicine reviews, 10*(6), 381-398.

Elizabeth Anderson, G. S. (2013). Effects of Exercise and Physical Activity on Anxiety. *Frontiers in Psychiatry, 4*.

Eric Konofal, M. L.-C. (2004). Iron Deficiency in Children With Attention-Deficit/Hyperactivity Disorder. *Archives of Pediatrics & Adolescent Medicine, 158*(12), 1113.

Genevieve Young, J. C. (2005). Omega-3 fatty acids and neuropsychiatric disorders. *Reproduction Nutrition Development, 45*(1), 1-28.

Hechtman, L. (2008). Treatment of adults with attention-deficit/hyperactivity disorder. *Neuropsychiatric Disease and Treatment*, 389.

Joel T. Nigg, A. L. (2015). Variation in an Iron Metabolism Gene Moderates the Association Between Blood Lead Levels and Attention-

Deficit/Hyperactivity Disorder in Children. *Psychological Science, 27*(2), 257-269.

K. Lindstrom, F. L. (2011). Preterm Birth and Attention-Deficit/Hyperactivity Disorder in Schoolchildren. *Pediatrics, 127*(5), 858-865.

Mats Johnson, S. Ö. (2009). Omega-3/Omega-6 Fatty Acids for Attention Deficit Hyperactivity Disorder. *Journal of Attention Disorders, 12*(5).

Megan R. McDougall, D. A. (2006). Having a Co-Twin With Attention-Deficit Hyperactivity Disorder. *Twin Research and Human Genetics, 9*(1), 148-154.

Natali Golan, E. S. (2004). Sleep disorders and daytime sleepiness in children with attention-deficit/hyperactive disorder. *Sleep, 27*(2), 261-266.

Nigel M. Williams, I. Z. (2010). Rare chromosomal deletions and duplications in attention-deficit hyperactivity disorder: a genome-wide analysis. *The Lancet, 376*(9750), 1401-1408.

Philip Shaw, M. G. (2007). Polymorphisms of the Dopamine D4 Receptor, Clinical Outcome, and Cortical Structure in Attention-Deficit/Hyperactivity Disorder. *Archives of General Psychiatry, 64*(8), 921.

Rosalind J. Neuman, E. L.-W. (2007). Prenatal Smoking Exposure and Dopaminergic Genotypes Interact to Cause a Severe ADHD Subtype. *Biological Psychiatry, 61*(12), 1320-1328.

Ruff, M. E. (2005). Attention Deficit Disorder and Stimulant Use: An Epidemic of Modernity. *Clinical Pediatrics, 44*(7), 557-563.

Samuele Cortese, E. K.-C. (2006). Sleep and alertness in children with attention-deficit/hyperactivity disorder: a systematic review of the literature. *Sleep, 29*(4), 504-511.

ADHD Workbook for Adults

Skills to Improve Concentration, Organization, Stress Management in Difficult Situations: Including Work, School, and Personal Relationships

Gerald Paul Clifford

© Copyright 2020 by Gerald Paul Clifford. All right reserved.

The work contained herein has been produced with the intent to provide relevant knowledge and information on the topic on the topic described in the title for entertainment purposes only. While the author has gone to every extent to furnish up to date and true information, no claims can be made as to its accuracy or validity as the author has made no claims to be an expert on this topic. Notwithstanding, the reader is asked to do their own research and consult any subject matter experts they deem necessary to ensure the quality and accuracy of the material presented herein.

This statement is legally binding as deemed by the Committee of Publishers Association and the American Bar Association for the territory of the United States. Other jurisdictions may apply their own legal statutes. Any reproduction, transmission, or copying of this material contained in this work without the express written consent of the copyright holder shall be deemed as a copyright violation as per the current legislation in force on the date of publishing and the subsequent time thereafter. All additional works derived from this material may be claimed by the holder of this copyright.

The data, depictions, events, descriptions, and all other information forthwith are considered to be true, fair, and accurate unless the work is expressly described as a work of fiction. Regardless of the nature of this work, the Publisher is exempt from any responsibility of actions taken by the reader in conjunction with this work. The Publisher acknowledges that the reader acts of their own accord and releases the author and Publisher of any responsibility for the observance of tips, advice, counsel, strategies, and techniques that may be offered in this volume.

Table of Contents

Introduction 7
Chapter 1: Understanding ADHD 11

What Is ADHD? 11
Why Does ADHD Happen? 12
Types of ADHD 14
What Is Adult ADHD? 15
ADHD Diagnosis in Adults 17
What Challenges Are Faced By Adults Who Have ADHD? 20

Chapter 2: Characteristics of ADHD 26

Distractibility and Difficulty to Concentrate 26
Impulsivity 28
Hyperactivity 29
Exaggerated Emotions... 30
Gender and ADHD... 33

Chapter 3: Making Time for Mindfulness and Exercise 37

Is Mindfulness Effective for ADHD? 38
Exercise and ADHD 43
Common Types of Exercises That Help Alleviate the Symptoms of ADHD 46

Chapter 4: How Can You Minimize the Triggers? 51

Some Common Triggers to be Aware of 51

Food Additives 51
Mineral Deficiencies 52
Stress 53
Poor Sleep 54
Technology 55

Tips for Minimizing Triggers 56

Maintain a Balanced Diet 56
Exercise Regularly 57
Work On Your Time Management Skills 57
Spend Time Outdoors 59
Get Enough Sleep 59

Chapter 5: Behavioral Therapy for ADHD ... 62

How Does Behavioral Therapy Work? 62
CBT for Adults 64

What Is CBT? 64
How Does CBT Help ADHD Adults? 67

What Is DBT? 74

Chapter 6: A Step-by-Step Guide to Become More Productive With ADHD 75

Step 1 - Don't Try Multitasking 75
Step 2 - Be Realistic 78
Step 3 – Stop Trying to be Perfect 79
Step 4 – Prep Your Environment 81
Step 5 – Time Your Tasks 84
Step 6 – Do the Fun Stuff First 85
Step 7 – Use Visual Reminders 86

Chapter 7: Treating ADHD With Medication 88

Stimulant Medications 90
Non-Stimulant Medications 96
When Should I Take Medications?......................... 99

Chapter 8: Dealing With ADHD Shame 104

What Is Shame? 104
Consequences of Shame 108
How to Silence the Haters? 110
How to Heal Shame? 113
Practice Self-Love 115

Chapter 9: ADHD and Relationships 121

What Is the Impact of ADHD on Relationships? . 121
Tips for a Healthier Relationship 125

Conclusion 128
Resources 133

Introduction

Congratulations on purchasing *ADHD Workbook for Adults,* and thank you for doing so.

In this book, you will find every detail that you need to know about ADHD and then learn the techniques with the help of which you can make your life easier. There are strategies that will help you identify ADHD in a person. Finding out that you have ADHD is one of the first steps towards recovering from the problem. The earlier you identify the disorder, the sooner you will get the treatment, and the faster you will be able to bring your life back on track.

Some of the most common symptoms of ADHD include disorganization, impulsivity, distractibility, and so on, and you are going to learn about all of these symptoms in detail in this book. One of the most common results of having ADHD is that both your personal and professional life is severely hampered. In the case of adults, they often cruise along with life, and eventually, they arrive at a stage when everything seems to be going wrong and falling apart. That is when they are diagnosed with ADHD.

Most people don't understand how frustrating ADHD can be. It is not only contradictory but also confusing. When people have to spend their day-to-day lives with this condition, it easily gets overwhelming. When you go to a specialist for diagnosis, they will ask you a lot of questions, and they will also provide you with a checklist of symptoms that you can go through. Medication alone is never enough to help you cope with the symptoms. You always need more, and by more, I mean that you need to take the help of therapy.

Most of us think that ADHD means a kid who is bouncing on the couch and running wildly around the house. But is that the only type of ADHD that you need to be aware of? No, because ADHD can happen to adults too, and that is not how it looks. In fact, there are several adults with ADHD who are not hyperactive, but they have other symptoms. Some people believe that ADHD is one of the most over-diagnosed conditions, but whether that is true or not, you have to understand that the implications on the life of the person are immense. They cannot keep up with their personal relationships, and they forget about stuff very easily. They make impulsive decisions and might go on a shopping spree all of a sudden just because they feel like it, or they might shift between jobs every month. But more often than not, these people are not particularly happy about the decisions they are taking and so, they regret it later. Their patterns and actions are mostly very self-destructive, and they easily fall into the clutches of depression ad addiction. The effort and struggle that has to be given by an ADHD individual are way more than anyone else who is doing the same thing.

We are not only going to break several myths surrounding ADHD, but we are also going to learn about several tactics that can help you cope with your symptoms and lead a more organized life. I know that maintaining a healthy routine can be your biggest nightmare when you have ADHD but trust me, with the proven strategies mentioned here, you are going to learn a lot of self-control and make a lot of improvement with routines.

I am sure that your doctor is going to suggest some medications for this, but that will not be enough. So, in order to get your priorities straight and getting things organized, you will need the help of a therapist. Whenever it comes to making a choice that needs to be made after considerable thought, it's best if you take a time out and then negotiate. If there are any negative feelings inside you, then they have to be removed by someone you trust in order to be able to make your recovery faster. You need this help, even more, when you think that you have not been able to keep up with the expectations of others.

Another thing to keep in mind is that just because someone is energetic and always enthusiastic about stuff, you cannot predict them to have ADHD. You will always find people who are not the quiet type, and they cannot seem to focus their mind on any one thing. So, they keep changing their focus from time to time. But that doesn't make them a patient of ADHD. In this book, you will learn many such facts about ADHD that are not that well-known among people, and that is what creates so much confusion. I am sure that all of you must have come across family members and friends who were all ready to give you advice on what ADHD is and how it can be cured. But most of them are unknown to what ADHD really is. So, before taking any advice from others, I suggest you read this book and consult a specialist for proper diagnosis.

I would also like to give you a small piece of advice here – don't try to finish this book in a rush. I know that most of you would want to finish it in a week. I know that you are also going to feel a sense of accomplishment once you finish this book, but if you want to truly get something out of this, then you need to learn the strategies by heart. And for that, you need to give this some time. It would help if you blocked time in your calendar with the intention of actually doing some work on your problem while reading this book. You have to remind yourself why you are doing this – it is because you want to. If you want change – a change that is going to stay – then you also need to put in the effort. Remind yourself that you deserve, and that is why you have undertaken this journey. And soon, you will see that with these skills under your belt, navigating through life has become so much easier.

There is no end to the number of books on this subject that you will get in the market, but I am thankful that you chose this one. I have tried my best to explain every detail in the most concise manner possible, and so I hope you enjoy it!

Chapter 1: Understanding ADHD

ADHD is a very common disorder. More than 10 million cases of ADHD are recorded in India per year. Here we will discuss the disorder in detail about the cause of this disorder, types, diagnosis, challenges faced by people suffering from this disorder, etc.

What Is ADHD?

The full form of this acronym is Attention-Deficit Hyperactivity Disorder. Out of all the people in the U.S, approximately 4.4% of the adult population is affected by this disorder which is mainly neurological in origin. It is more likely to occur to men than to women. 5.4 percent of men are diagnosed with ADHD, whereas 3.2 percent of women are diagnosed with ADHD. It is a disorder that causes a deficiency of attention and causes heightened levels of impulsive and hyperactive behaviors. Patients who have ADHD have low persistence, face difficulty in focusing on a particular thing, and are disorganized. They are always restless and find extreme difficulty in being calm. They often tend to make impulsive decisions because of the hyperactivity, which may end up proving to be harmful to them.

Earlier, ADHD was considered to be just a childhood condition, but now it is accepted to be an adulthood condition as well. The rates of persistence of ADHD vary from 6 percent to 30 percent. The persistence rates can be even higher, too.

Studies have shown that in the last decade, there is a hike in the rate of ADHD diagnosis among adults in the U.S. (Winston Chung, 2019)

Why Does ADHD Happen?

Though the exact causes of ADHD are still unknown, there are certain factors that definitely play a part in the development of this disorder. Let us see some of those factors.

- *Hereditary:* ADHD can be inherited. If your parent suffers from this disorder, you have a risk of inheriting the same. Certain genetic characteristics pass down through the generation. You have a more than 50 percent chance of developing this disorder if your parent has it, and you have more than 30 percent chance of developing this disorder if your older sibling has it. However, the inheritance of ADHD is way more complex, so it is not just because of a single genetic fault.

- *Pregnancy Problems:* ADHD may also develop from certain pregnancy-related problems. A child who is born premature, or is born slightly underweight, has a higher risk of developing this disorder. A child whose mother has had difficult pregnancies earlier is also prone to develop this disorder. The frontal lobe of your brain is responsible for controlling emotions and impulses. So, children having head injuries in this region are at a greater risk of developing this disorder. Pregnant women who drink alcohol or smoke are at a higher risk of giving birth to a child having ADHD. Getting exposed to pesticides, PCBs, or leads, while pregnancy may also increase the chance of the baby developing ADHD.

- *Brain Functions:* After birth, if a child develops some infectious disorder that may affect the brain tissues, like encephalitis or meningitis, then that may affect the working ways of sending signals. This may also induce symptoms of ADHD. Sugar and certain food additives are often considered to induce ADHD. However, researches show that ADHD has got nothing to do with dietary factors.

Chemicals present in the brain, also known as neurotransmitters, work differently in adults and children having ADHD. Even the working ways of the nerve pathways tend to differ. Certain areas of the brain of children having ADHD are smaller or less active than those children who don't have this disorder. The neurotransmitter dopamine also plays a significant role. It is linked to learning, attention, mood, sleep, and movement.

Researches have shown differences in brain activities in people with ADHD and without ADHD. The exact significance is still not clear.

- *Other Factors:* Few groups of people are believed to be at a higher risk of developing ADHD like people who were born premature, i.e., before the thirty-seventh week of pregnancy. People with epilepsy are also prone to develop ADHD. People with brain damage also tend to develop ADHD. This damage can occur either in the mother's womb or can also occur because of a serious injury in the head later in life.

Types of ADHD

ADHD is characterized by hyperactivity, impulsivity, and inattention. Most of the people who don't have ADHD also experience a certain degree of impulsive or inattentive behavior, but people with ADHD experience severe hyperactivity-impulsiveness and inattentiveness. There are three types of ADHD, and each type of ADHD is linked to one or more characteristics. They are as follows:

- *Predominantly Inattentive ADHD*: People suffering from this type of ADHD mostly have symptoms of inattention. Their impulsive nature or hyperactivity is not as much as their inattentiveness. Although, at times, it is possible that they have to struggle with hyperactivity or impulse control, but they are not the main characteristics of predominantly inattentive ADHD. This type of ADHD is more common in girls than in boys.

- *Predominantly Hyperactive-Impulsive ADHD:* People who have predominantly hyperactive-impulsive ADHD have symptoms of impulsivity and hyperactivity more than the symptoms of inattention. Patients having predominantly hyperactive-impulsive ADHD may also be inattentive at times, but that is certainly not the main characteristic of this disorder. Children suffering from this disorder can cause a lot of disturbance in their school's classroom. They make learning way more difficult for other students as well as themselves.

- *Combination ADHD:* If a person has combination ADHD, then it means their symptoms don't exactly fall under hyperactive-impulsive behavior or inattention. Instead, they experience a combination of symptoms of both categories.

What Is Adult ADHD?

Being an adult, balancing everything in your life can be really hectic. If you see that you are constantly forgetful, disorganized, clumsy, late, and always struggling to meet your responsibilities, then it is possible that you have ADHD. ADHD, in adults, can cause a lot of hindrance in both their personal and professional life. If you were diagnosed with ADHD at childhood, then it is possible that you carry those symptoms with you into your adulthood as well. It is also possible that you get diagnosed with ADHD in your adulthood, but while you were a child, you were never diagnosed with ADHD. It is possible for ADHD to remain undiagnosed in childhood. In earlier days, not many people were aware of it. Children having the symptoms of ADHD were mostly termed as troublemakers, slackers, dreamers, etc. in the earlier days, which is why chances of ADHD being undiagnosed were very much high at that time.

When you were a child, you may have been able to compensate for those symptoms of ADHD. But when you grow up, it is not that easy to run away from your responsibilities. When you are a grown-up individual, you are expected to run a household, raise a family, pursue a lucrative career, and many more. These responsibilities demand concentration, calmness, and focus, which become very difficult for an ADHD patient to maintain. Even normal people find it difficult to meet up to all these responsibilities. So, for people with ADHD, this is just straight away impossible. The only good thing about this disorder is that it is treatable. With the help of a little creativity, support, and education, you can be able to overcome the symptoms of ADHD. You can even turn some of your biggest weaknesses into your strengths. Being an adult, it is totally possible for you to fight against this disorder and succeed.

The symptoms of this disorder are mostly noticed at a young age. The symptoms become more clear and evident when the child's circumstances happen to change. For example, when they start to go to school, they show clear symptoms of ADHD. Most of the cases are diagnosed when the children are mostly between 6 to 12 years of age. ADHD symptoms generally improve with age, but there are many people who were diagnosed with ADHD in childhood and still continue to face problems when they are adults. Inattentiveness and restlessness do not always mean that you have ADHD, but it's a possibility. So, you should never ignore these things and should get a proper diagnosis.

ADHD Diagnosis in Adults

ADHD diagnosis in adults is way more difficult than that in kids. The main reason is the presence of varied opinions of whether the symptoms list used to diagnose ADHD in children should also be implied while diagnosing ADHD in adults or not. In some situations, an adult exhibiting five or more symptoms of impulsiveness and hyperactivity, or five or more of inattentiveness symptoms, may be diagnosed with ADHD, as listed in the children's ADHD diagnostic criteria. The specialist must ask you questions about the present symptoms. According to the current diagnostic guideline, ADHD in adults can't be confirmed if the symptoms were not present since childhood. In case you find difficulties in remembering the problems you faced as a child, the clinician may ask your parents, closed ones, or even check your old school records to search for any abnormality that you possessed as a child. In order to get diagnosed with ADHD, an adult must have certain effects on different areas of life. If the adult faces problems in difficulty in maintaining relationships with their partner and family, or if he faces difficulty in keeping and making friends, or if he tends to drive his car very roughly, then he is likely to have ADHD. If your problems are recent and not repetitive and old, then you are not going to get diagnosed with ADHD.

Most of the criteria that are used for diagnosing ADHD in adults are mainly focused on the identification of symptoms in children and teens. So, there are higher chances of misdiagnosis in adults. In order to perform a proper diagnosis of ADHD patients, the physicians must know the nuances of ADHD and must also be aware of the overlapping conditions developed in adulthood. Earlier doctors believed that ADHD is a disorder that only children could have, but with time, it is clearly evident that a lot of adults are facing the symptoms of ADHD later in life and are seeking an evaluation in their adulthood. So, the understanding of ADHD diagnosis has improved quite a lot in the last few decades. Most people try to compensate for the symptoms of ADHD in their own way. These undiagnosed ADHD patients often try to fight inattentiveness, impulsiveness, and hyperactivity because they are good problem solvers, creative, and bright. But when they are overwhelmed with continuous increasing challenges and responsibilities, that is when reality kicks in, and they seek medical help. According to a certified adult psychiatrist, the average age of ADHD diagnosis is 39 in his practice.

There is a symptom guide to diagnose ADHD in children, but there is no such guide or manual to diagnose ADHD in adults. The only way of successful diagnosis of ADHD in adults is to run a thorough clinical interview to obtain a detailed medical history. It is imperative that the patient goes to a clinician who is particularly specialized in ADHD. This is to make sure that the clinician will take out time to gather all the required information from you in order to diagnose ADHD in adulthood. The clinical interview may also incorporate neurophysiological testing in order to obtain greater insight into the subject's weaknesses and strengths. This will help to identify any comorbid or co-existing conditions.

Most of the physicians miss out on the differential diagnosis. ADHD symptoms often are the results of different mental health issues like a mood disorder or anxiety. The clinician must have a thorough understanding of the comorbid conditions. The emotional sensitivity resulting from ADHD may also appear as mere anxiety or a mood disorder. It is the duty of the clinician to understand how these symptoms can mimic each other and at what point they differ; otherwise, you will just end up wasting energy, time, and money. A clinician who is trained in just one of these conditions may end up making the wrong diagnosis. So, the clinician must have proper knowledge of ADHD and everything associated with it in order to perform a successful diagnosis of his or her patients. In order to find a good clinician, it is advised that you go to a directory who will guide you about whom you should pursue. Physicians who have no experience of performing mental health diagnoses must refer their patients to a psychologist or psychiatrist having relevant experience of diagnosing ADHD patients.

What Challenges Are Faced By Adults Who Have ADHD?

Adult ADHD has a massive impact on one's life. If it remains ineffectively treated, untreated, or undiagnosed, it can have adverse effects on the quality of life led by a person and psychological well-being.

- *Career Challenges:* ADHD symptoms like forgetfulness, procrastination, poor concentration, and poor time management may make maintaining a healthy life at the workplace and school very much difficult. Many studies have shown that people having ADHD suffers tremendously in their school life and workplace (Aparajita B. Kuriyan, 2012). Studies have shown that people suffering from

ADHD who did not receive proper treatment at childhood faces extreme difficulty in maintaining and gaining employment compared to other people (Anne Halmøy, 2009). They feel a constant sense of underachievement and faces difficulty in following corporate rules, following a 9 to 5 routine, and maintaining deadlines. Another big problem is finances. People having ADHD are prone to have difficulties in financial management, as well. They struggle with due debt, late fees, lost paperwork, unpaid bills, etc. because of impulsive spending.

- *Relationship Problems:* Symptoms of ADHD like impulsivity, inefficiency to follow tasks, low frustration tolerance, and poor listening skills tend to have a detrimental impact on social connections, familial relationships, friendships, and romantic relationships (Ylva Ginsberg, 2014). You may feel tired because of the constant nagging of your loved ones for you to put yourself together. People close to you may feel hurt because of your insensitivity and irresponsibility. The effects of ADHD may lead to loss of confidence, disappointment, hopelessness, frustration, and embarrassment. You can get a feeling as if you can never get a hold of your life and live up to your fullest potential, leaving you with low self-esteem. You tend to hurt your loved one's expectations, ending up hurting them as well as yourself for not being able to meet their expectations.

- *Criminal Tendencies:* Certain researches have linked adult ADHD to rule-breaking, criminality, and other safety and legal issues, which includes a heightened chance of getting into car accidents as compared to other people without ADHD (Zheng Chang, 2017). Certain studies also show that individuals exhibiting ADHD symptoms are more likely to get engaged in various criminal activities compared to other people. A recent study showed that 26 percent of prisoners have adult ADHD (Stéphanie Baggio, 2018).

It is seen that men who had childhood ADHD are 2 to 3 times more likely to be incarcerated, convicted, or arrested in their adulthood compared to those who don't have ADHD. The impulsivity that lies within the people suffering from ADHD impairs their ability to control emotions, behavior, and thoughts. Their self-regulating capability is also damaged. A study showed that there is a link between criminal behavior and impaired self-control (Alexander T. Vazsonyi, 2017).

Children suffering from ODD (Oppositional Defiant Disorder) portray a very disobedient, hostile, defiant, and negative behavior towards the authorities and parents. They often show resentful, vindictive, and angry behavior. They grow up and gradually tend to incline towards various criminal activities. 25 to 75 percent of people having ADHD also have ODD.

- *Substance Abuse Tendencies:* Substance abuse and adult ADHD are strongly linked. Substance Use Disorder or SUD is very common in patients with ADHD than those who have not been diagnosed with this disorder. In fact, it is two times more likely to happen to ADHD patients. Many adults suffering from ADHD and having a SUD report uses drugs and alcohol to manage ADHD symptoms and self-medicate.

- *Comorbid Disorder:* 60 to 70 percent of people suffering from adult ADHD have a comorbid disorder. According to a study on adult ADHD, about 15 percent of them were found to have a substance abuse disorder diagnosis, 50 percent of them were found to have anxiety disorder diagnosis, and 40 percent of them were diagnosed with a mood disorder (Benjamín Piñeiro-Dieguez, 2016).

- *Health Issues:* ADHD symptoms can also contribute to a wide range of health problems like chronic tension, stress, substance abuse, compulsive eating, etc. People suffering from ADHD often tend to forget to take vital medicines, skip doctor's appointments, ignore medical instructions, neglect vital checkups, and thus are more likely to get themselves into trouble.

If you suffer from ADHD, then that might not be the only health issue you have. ADHD often brings other health issues along with it. Adults suffering from ADHD may have health issues due to alcohol and drugs, sleep problems, depression, etc.

- *Depression:* ADHD is very much likely to make you feel frustrated and sad at times. Clinical depression is very much different than just being sad. It is way more severe and causes the day to day problems in social activities, relationships, school, work, etc. 70 percent of the people who have ADHD get treated for depression at some point in their life.

- *Sleep Problems:* Problems with sleep cycles are very common in people who have ADHD. Even kids with ADHD find it difficult to obtain enough rest. People with ADHD are two to three times more likely to have sleep problems than those who don't have ADHD.

- *Serious Behavioral Problems:* People with ADHD often develop ODD (Oppositional Defiant Disorder). In this, people tend to resentment and anger without any proper reason. They often have a tendency to blame others for their own bad behavior. They purposely annoy people and tend to break the rules and argue with everyone.

Another behavioral disorder noticed in people with ADHD is CD (Conduct Disorder). ODD often turns into CD and becomes more severe. Forty-five percent of teens who have ADHD tend to develop CD later in their life, and 25 percent of children suffering from ADHD also develop CD later in their life. People with CD tend to skip school, steal, destroy properties, and shows extreme aggressive behavior towards animals and people.

Chapter 2: Characteristics of ADHD

In the previous chapter, I already told you about the different types of ADHD that are there. But the symptoms of ADHD fall into two main categories which are –

- Impulsiveness and hyperactivity
- Inattentiveness

There are some people who have symptoms from both categories while there are others who face only one of them. In this chapter, we are going to talk about the characteristics of ADHD in detail. But remember that you are not to use the information mentioned in this chapter for performing self-diagnosis. You can, however, refer to the information in order to figure out for certain whether your problem needs special attention or not. Once you visit a specialist, he/she will be able to diagnose the problem to be ADHD or something else.

Distractibility and Difficulty to Concentrate

Distractibility will, no doubt, be one of the biggest barriers in your path when you are trying to deal with ADHD. But first, let us explore what the term 'distractibility' truly means. It means that you don't have the ability to steer clear of visual distractions or any other unimportant distractions and do the task that you have been assigned. For example, there are several adults with ADHD who simply cannot work when there is the slightest noise in their surroundings – it can be something as simple as someone's footsteps. In short, when people have ADHD, they sort of do not know how to filter out the distractions. So, when there are too many things happening in their surroundings, all of that automatically starts competing for her attention.

When a person with ADHD experiences this feeling of distractibility, they cannot usually frame it in words. This is mainly because they themselves do not understand it that well. People often see them as space cadets or airheads. In fact, when ADHD goes unnoticed or undiagnosed until adulthood, people who struggle with distractibility often think that they are scatterbrained and that it cannot possibly be a part of any disorder. That is why it is so important that you address the problem of distractibility separately in your treatment plan because it is definitely one of the most overwhelming parts of suffering from ADHD.

Another thing to note here is that distractibility is not a symptom that is present at all times in the patient. For example, if a person is being attended to individually, he/she might remain focused and not be distracted.

Impulsivity

Impulsivity is one of those symptoms of ADHD that people often ignore. Being impulsive doesn't only mean that the person has zero sense of self-discipline or is rude. There is much more to it than just that. Impulsiveness comes from changes in the brain's signaling system, which is impacted in a person with ADHD. So, a person takes random actions without thinking it through. They completely overlook the consequences that their actions are going to have. They simply act on a whim. So, an adult with ADHD might answer people rudely all of a sudden or scream because they are angry.

The different parts of the brain are responsible for different activities. Similarly, it is your thalamus that is responsible for impulse control. Its function is very similar to that of a gate because it is the thalamus that decides which signals it is going to stop and which it is going to allow. So, if a signal comes along that is a red flag, the frontal cortex is made known of it by the thalamus with the help of the limbic-hippocampal connections. The frontal cortex of the brain is the region that is responsible for solving problems and handling your expression of different emotions. But when someone has ADHD, the gate of the thalamus does not function the way it normally should. So, they face difficulty in holding back their words even when they know that what they are going to say might hurt someone badly. This is also why ADHD adults go on a shopping spree from time to time because they cannot put a rein on their money-spending impulses.

It is because of impulsiveness that people act at the spur of the moment. You can also say that these people do not have a good sense of judgment and very poor planning skills. Gradually, they become disorganized and disorderly. The symptom of distractibility, along with impulsiveness, is what makes these people so untidy with cluttered work desks, unpaid bills, untucked shirts, missed deadlines, and careless writing style. Another part of this impulsiveness is antisocial behavior.

Hyperactivity

The characteristics of hyperactivity are more commonly noticed in children than in adults. Even when it comes to adults, you will find that it is men who display this symptom more than women. This symptom refers to the behavior of constant fidgeting and the need to move. Some people have the habit of shuffling their feet or continuously tapping their fingers even while they are in the middle of a conversation. There are different ways in which the symptom of hyperactivity can manifest itself. But you have to keep in mind that when people grow old, hyperactivity is the first symptom that dies down, and so, you cannot identify or diagnose ADHD solely based on hyperactivity. In any case, if someone is suffering from a problem of hyperactivity, they will not be able to sit in a single place for a long time. They will also not prefer doing quiet activities and have a knack towards energetic activities.

Exaggerated Emotions

Emotions are often heightened in adults who have ADHD. The root cause of this characteristic also lies in the brain. Adult ADHD often causes people to get flooded by a certain emotion all of a sudden, even though that emotion was only momentary. This is mainly because of some problems in the working memory. Unfortunately, the system of diagnosis, that is currently followed for ADHD, doesn't factor in exaggerated emotions or emotional challenges. But if we are to follow the research-based evidence, then we'll see, then it is shown that people with ADHD have a hot temper, impatience, a very low tolerance level to frustration, and excitability.

These challenges that we are talking about also find their origin in the human brain. In usual scenarios, anyone who has ADHD won't seem that much affected by someone's feelings or actions and would appear to be completely unaware. But there are times when these emotions become exaggerated because of impairments. Our emotions are relayed through various signals in the brain, and in people with ADHD, these networks do not function the way they should and are somewhat limited.

So, if something is denied to the adult, they often get filled with rage and cannot keep their anger under control even when the issue is not that important. Thus, they end up giving an extreme response to something very insignificant. This phenomenon is also known as flooding because the emotion at that point of time has taken up all the space inside his/her head. It is very similar to a virus attack on your laptop, where the laptop does not function properly because the virus takes up the entire hard disk. So, the person starts focusing on that one single emotion and overlooks everything else. They cannot take in any information that is given to them at that moment. That is why any attempt to regulate or reduce their anger doesn't work out.

Another example of having exaggerated emotions is that people with ADHD are very sensitive to any kind of disapproval. That one salient emotion becomes so superior in their minds that they cannot focus on anything else. So, let us say some coworker has disapproved the patient's idea on a project. Even though the disapproval was done in a very polite manner, the patient might think of it as extreme criticism, and they would right away go into a self-defense mode. Their outburst at that moment would be so huge that anyone would think something grave has happened. Only if the patient had been listening to his/her carefully, they would have been able to understand that it was not a criticism at all.

Adults who have ADHD also face a lot of social anxiety that they keep bottled up inside themselves. They are constantly in this cycle of self-loathing because they feel that they are uncool, unappealing, and not competent enough like everyone around them. This can be really toxic and make life even more difficult for an ADHD patient.

At other times, people with ADHD do understand the emotion, but they are too scared to deal with them. Their tolerance level for those emotions is too low. Whenever something gets serious or is too painful to talk about, it overwhelms them, and so they avoid the topic altogether. This doesn't help in any way to solve the problem. Such behaviors are often noticed when ADHD adults have to be in a social gathering with a bunch of people they don't know or when there are plenty of deadlines knocking on the door.

The ADHD brain is mostly incapable of seeing minor problems and dangerous threats separately, and so, their emotions are always wrong. So, even when a situation does not require them to panic, they start panicking. It is somewhat uncontrollable for them because their brain is wired in such a way. So, an adult having ADHD cannot deal with stressful events, and they cannot behave realistically. When they have to make a decision, thinking rationally seems a big deal to them.

Another example of exaggerated emotions in ADHD adults is that many of them suffer from dysthymia, especially when their ADHD goes untreated for a long duration of time. Dysthymia is characterized by sadness, and it is a mood disorder that often happens over the long term. When the right treatment is not received, adults with ADHD have to deal with a lot of negativity and frustrations in their day-to-day life, and that is what leads to this mood disorder. These people are also seen to have a very poor sense of self-esteem, and their energy levels are always very low.

Every action that we take in our lives is motivated by our emotions. So, when ADHD is either not diagnosed or not treated properly in adults, they often seek immediate gratification, and for this, they pursue only those activities that can give them that. That is why, in the long term, they fail to provide a consistent effort to those tasks whose rewards are going to be realized at a later time. Moreover, there have been several brain imaging studies done on ADHD patients that show that the ADHD brain does not identify satisfaction or pleasure like that of a normal brain, especially for tasks whose rewards are delayed.

Gender and ADHD

In this section, we are going to talk about the characteristics of ADHD with respect to gender. This topic is often overlooked. According to statistics, ADHD is more commonly diagnosed in boys than that in girls, and this disparity has nothing to do with ADHD affecting boys more than girls. This is not an explanation. The more plausible explanation is that the symptoms manifest themselves in different ways in girls and boys. The symptoms in girls are more subtle, and so, people often tend to miss them out.

In research, it has been found that impulsivity and always trying to move and such externalized symptoms are more common in boys (Rucklidge, 2010). On the contrary, in the case of girls, the symptoms are internalized. They have a very poor sense of self-esteem, and they are always inattentive. Another significant difference is that physical aggression is not something that is commonly seen in girls. It is seen in boys, whereas, in girls, it is verbal aggression that is common. But the fact that symptoms in girls are often overlooked means that they are undiagnosed and, thus, left untreated for a very long time. When they move into adulthood and are diagnosed with ADHD, the disorder has already jeopardized their self-esteem to a great extent in all those years. In the case of boys, whenever they feel that their frustration is becoming too much to handle, they take it out externally, but girls, on the other hand, don't do that. They direct their frustration and anger inward and keep blaming themselves for everything. Thus, ADHD in girls leads to some other problems as well, for example, eating disorders and depression.

In 2012, it was found in research that tendency to self-harm and commit suicides is much higher in those girls who are suffering from combined-type ADHD (Stephen P. Hinshaw, 2012). They also mentioned that this tendency stayed despite the fact that symptoms of impulsiveness and hyperactivity had subsided in 40% of them by the time they reached adolescence.

Now that you know that the common symptoms that we talked about at the beginning of this chapter are not usually as prominent in girls, how will you identify that they have ADHD? Well, there are some symptoms that you should keep an eye on, and they are as follows -

- Anxiety
- No or very low sense of self-esteem
- Withdrawn from daily life
- Inability to focus
- Always daydreaming or inattentive
- Poor academic record
- Impairment of intellectuality
- Signs of verbal aggressions in petty situations (name-calling, taunting, teasing, etc.)
- Not listening to others

The most common question that everyone has after learning about this difference in boys and girls is whether the treatment process is different for these genders. Well, the treatment is the same. But whenever someone goes to a doctor, he/she will consider your individual differences because not everyone has the same response, and not everyone has the same behavioral symptoms. So, a particular combination of therapy and medication is fixed for each and every person depending upon their needs.

Chapter 3: Making Time for Mindfulness and Exercise

Attention deficit hyperactivity disorder (ADHD) can show up at different stages of life and in several ways. It happens due to the differences in the brain, which affects important functioning skills like memory, attention, impulsiveness, concentration, and more. For a majority of children and adults suffering from ADHD, maintaining self-regulation and paying attention are two of the persistent daily challenges that they have to face. So, it can be said that a natural remedy for ADHD would be some kind of attention training that helps hone their self-control. It would be incredibly powerful and invaluable.

While the symptoms of ADHD can be managed by therapy and meditation, they are not the only options. According to studies, another good way to improve your focus and calm your mind is through mindfulness meditation. Mindfulness or mindful meditation is a part of several religious traditions like Buddhism. However, it is not necessarily spiritual or religious. It consists of developing a greater awareness of everything that is happening around you every moment by paying close attention to your bodily sensations, feelings, and thoughts. It can also be used as a tool to promote psychological well-being. According to a survey conducted by *ADDitude* magazine in 2017, more than 1/3rd of adults suffering from ADHD use mindfulness, and almost forty percent of them have given it high ratings.

Is Mindfulness Effective for ADHD?

Just like exercises can help strengthen a specific weak muscle in your body, the same thing can also be true for your brain. Mindfulness helps enhance your capacity to control your attention. It allows you to focus on yourself and teaches you how to observe yourself. In addition to that, when you get distracted, mindfulness trains you to bring back your wandering mind to the present moment.

Unlike other treatments for ADHD, practicing mindfulness helps to develop your inner skills. It helps increase your ability to develop different kinds of relationships, to train your attention, and strengthen your ability to self-observe so that you can control your attention. Therefore, it makes you learn how to pay attention to paying attention so that you don't react impulsively and become aware of your emotional state. Meditation thickens the prefrontal cortex of your brain. The prefrontal cortex is the region of your brain that is involved in controlling your impulses, planning, and focusing. It also increases the level of dopamine in your brain, which gets decreased in people who have ADHD. Thus, it is believed that meditation helps people suffering from ADHD.

If you find long durations of sitting meditation to be very overwhelming, here are a few ways to help you get started.

- **Take a Class** – You can try signing up for a meditation class to harness the power of positive peer pressure. Following routines can be hard for people suffering from ADHD, and so it is hard for them to practice sitting down for a long period of time. Having a structure and group support can be helpful for them so that they don't feel like they are doing it alone. There are several centers that teach mindful meditation. Some centers provide 8-week programs that have weekly training sessions of 2.5 hours each along with at-home practice. They generally begin with seated meditations for 5 minutes every day at home and then work up to fifteen to twenty minutes. They also provide you with the option of practicing longer or replacing seated meditation with mindful walking. As some people who have ADHD tend to be better at learning visually, some centers also use visual aids such as a photo of a cloudy sky in order to describe the principle concepts. The clouds represent all the sensations, feelings, and thoughts that pass by, and the blue sky depicts an area of awareness.

However, your ADHD won't get much better if you do it for just a few minutes a day. Even though the meditation sessions are essential, the key is to be mindful of your actions throughout the day by being aware of where you are focused while you're performing your daily activities. For instance, you might notice that when you are behind the wheel, your attention often goes to the chores you need to do later that day. A majority of people follow mindfulness while eating. You can use the techniques of mindfulness anytime you begin to feel overwhelmed once you are accustomed to checking in with your mind and body.

- **Make it Your Own** – Individuals who have ADHD are encouraged to use mindfulness while performing their daily activities. You can even practice mindfulness on your own. Simply, choose a comfortable place where no one would disturb you and sit down and spend five minutes concentrating on the feelings of breathing in and breathing out. Concentrate on how you feel when your stomach rises and falls. In some time, you will begin to notice that your mind is wandering off to something else – your plans for the day or some noise you just heard or your job. Label these thoughts as "thinking" and put your attention back on your breath.

Try to perform this mental exercise every day. Increase the duration of time you spend on the mental training every couple of weeks – ten minutes, fifteen, up to twenty minutes, or even more if you want to. Try performing the same exercise every day and concentrate on your breath for some time as you are sitting in front of your computer, or when you are stopped at a red light, or when you are walking from one place to another. By doing this, you can eventually practice mindfulness at any moment, even while you are conversing with others. Turning on your state of mind-awareness any time during the day is a great exercise, even if it is only for a few minutes. You are essentially letting go of the busy-ness of your thoughts and bring your focus back to everything that is happening in the present moment in daily life.

- **Practice Self-Compassion** – People suffering from the challenges of ADHD for several years can be left with crippled self-esteem. You can learn to be more accepting of your weaknesses and strengths through self-compassion. Having an attitude of acceptance can also help improve and manage your areas of weaknesses. For instance, if you are more compassionate towards your problems with time management, then you don't have to pretend that you don't have a problem. You can get proactive about having the tools to manage your time properly without having to feel shameful every time you get late.

Studies examining the non-pharmacological interventions for individuals suffering from ADHD have increased in recent years and given several more treatment options for patients. Current empirical studies back the logic behind using mindfulness techniques to alleviate ADHD. They also provide promising basic-level support for suggesting the usefulness of mindfulness sessions (John T. Mitchell, 2015).

In one study, a mindfulness meditation program conducted in a group was administered to a sample of adolescents and adults with ADHD for eight weeks. Pre- and post-treatment assessments showed that there was an improvement in anxious, depressive, hyperactive-impulsive, and inattentive symptoms.

A study conducted in 2008 with eight adolescents and twenty-five adults, half of whom suffered from the combined type of ADHD (both hyperactive and inactive), revealed that the results were very promising. Significant improvements in both hyperactivity and inattention were observed through the study. The cognitive tests showed that the participants improved their ability to stay focused on one thing even when several other things were competing for their attention. It was also revealed that the majority of them felt less sad and stressed out when the study was completed.

Another study which came out in the *Journal of Child and Family Studies* in the year 2011 studied the outcome of a mindfulness-based training program that took place over the duration of eight weeks (Saskia van der Oord, 2011). The participants included children within the age of eight to twelve years, and a parallel mindful training was also being conducted for their parents. The study reported a significant decrease in the symptoms of ADHD, as were reported by the parents after the eight-week training program. There was also a decrease in over-reactivity and parental stress.

Exercise and ADHD

ADHD can affect both children as well as adults. It can make it difficult for adults to finish their tasks, control their emotions, and pay attention. Similar to children, adults are also given medications and stimulants to control their symptoms of ADHD. They also have therapy sessions that help them stay focused and get organized. Just like mindfulness meditation, exercise is another such method of treatment for ADHD that doesn't require a visit to a therapist's office or a prescription. Studies show that exercising regularly can improve the symptoms of ADHD in adults and also improve their thinking ability.

Studies have shown that exercise is not only good for toning muscles and shedding fat; it can also help you to keep your brain in good shape. Broad science says that exercise can help manage ADHD by increasing the release of neurotransmitters. Chemicals known as neurotransmitters are released by your brain when you exercise. These neurotransmitters include norepinephrine and dopamine, which helps with clear thinking and attention. Individuals suffering from ADHD tend to have a lesser amount of dopamine in their brains. The stimulants and medicines that are used for the treatment of ADHD in adults increase the level of dopamine available to the brain. Therefore, it can be said that a workout session can have similar effects like stimulant medications. Regular exercise can increase the baseline levels of norepinephrine and dopamine by increasing the development of several new receptors in specific regions of the brain.

It also helps to balance the level of norepinephrine in the arousal center located in the stem of the brain. The tone of the locus coeruleus is improved through chronic exercise. As a result of this, people are less prone to react out of proportion or get startled because of any given situation. They also fell less irritable. In the same way, exercise also administers the transmission fluids for the basal ganglia, which causes the smooth changes of the attention system. This region is an essential site for binding the stimulants, and brain scans also reveal that it is not normal in people suffering from ADHD.

Exercising can benefit other regions of the brain as well. For example, an overactive cerebellum can contribute to fidgetiness. According to several recent studies, these regions are brought back into balance by ADHD medications that can increase the levels of norepinephrine and dopamine. And when it comes to increasing the levels of norepinephrine, if the exercise is complex, it gets better.

Some of the benefits that exercise can provide for adults suffering from ADHD are:

- Improve the level of brain-derived neurotrophic factors that are involved in memory and learning. This protein is present in lesser amounts in people suffering from ADHD.

- Improves executive functions that are required to remember details, organize, and plan.

- Improves working memory

- Decreases compulsive behavior and improves impulse control

- Ease anxiety and stress

Any kinds of physical activities like skateboarding, whitewater paddling, mountain biking, rock climbing, gymnastics, ice skating, ballet, and martial arts are very good for adults suffering from ADHD. The technical movements that are used to perform these kinds of physical activities active a huge array of brain regions that help control intense focus and concentration, inhibition, fine motor adjustments, error connection, switching, evaluating consequences, sequencing, timing, and control balance. In the extreme, when you engage in these activities, it also becomes a matter of survival – preventing yourself from drowning in the swirling pool of whitewater, or hurting yourself on the balance beam, or avoiding a karate chop. Thus, it helps you to tap into the concentrating power of your mind's fight-or-flight response. You feel plenty of motivation to learn the techniques that are required for such activities when your mind is on high alert. For the brain, it would feel like a do or die situation. And, thus you will be in the aerobic range while taking part in these activities, which will make it easier for you to learn new strategies and moves and also boost your cognitive abilities.

Exercise also helps regulate the amygdale and has a good effect on the limbic system. In people with ADHD, the amygdale can help blunt the hair-trigger responsiveness that is experienced by several people and sends the reaction to another source of stimulus. This prevents you from going overboard and creating a scene out of anger.

Common Types of Exercises That Help Alleviate the Symptoms of ADHD

For a majority of patients, exercise is recommended as a method to help manage their symptoms of ADHD. Several studies have revealed that one of the best treatments for children and adults with ADHD is regular exercise. This is mainly because exercise helps them get rid of the extra raw energy present in their bodies in a healthy manner. Here are some of the common types of exercises that help alleviate the symptoms of ADHD:

- **Walking** – Walking is one of the simplest aerobic exercises that you can do. What's great about walking is that it can be done by almost anyone of any age group. All you require is a great pair of shoes. The benefits of walking doubles if you walk outdoors. Walking helps tone your leg muscles and also increases your heart rate. Children and adults suffering from ADHD can also benefit from being outside surrounded by greenery. A research conducted on children with ADHD revealed that even walking in the park for twenty minutes can help improve their concentration.

- **Dancing** – Many people suffering from ADHD find dance classes very appealing as a social form of exercise. The best kinds of dances are those that involve fast-paced movements that give you the opportunity to release all your extra energy. A research conducted in Sweden with boys aged five to seven found that participating in dance classes helped them to increase their concentration while doing their schoolwork and also helped to calm them down.

- **Swimming** – Swimming is another aerobic exercise that can help you tone your muscles and improve your heart rate. People suffering from ADHD can get a big boost from being in a swim team because even though they are part of a team, they have to perform individually. It might be hard for people suffering from ADHD to be a part of a sports team if they have to spend a lot of time just waiting for their turn to play. An individual sport like swimming can be a great exercise for this reason.

- **Yoga** – Yoga is extremely deliberate and slow, while people suffering from ADHD are extremely hyperactive. Research has revealed that yoga can be a good form of exercise for you, even if you are suffering from ADHD, because it helps you to focus on yourself. It teaches you to pay attention to your own body and concentrate on your breathing. It forces you to be in the present moment by becoming grounded. Doing yoga can thus help you learn how to concentrate and focus better.

- **Martial arts** – Different forms of martial arts like tai chi, aikido, tae-kwon-do, karate, etc. requires your full attention both mentally and physically. In addition to that, martial arts have a set of fixed rules which need to be followed. This helps add more structure to your everyday life. They can help you feel relaxed and focused at the same time, and this can help you alleviate your symptoms of ADHD. One of the most helpful martial arts is tai chi, as it is also a meditative practice. It can help boost your concentration skills and relieve your stress. Research has revealed that practicing tai chi regularly can help you develop higher levels of self-confidence and focus on other activities. You get trained in several skills like fine motor skills, consequences of actions, memory, timing, balance, focus, and concentration when you do martial arts.

- **Strength training** – You can go for aerobic exercises such as jogging, swimming, and walking first if you are just starting to exercise. You can add in some strength work after you have done simple aerobic exercises for a while in order to add some variety. You can try exercises like weightlifting, pull-ups, pushups, squats, lunges, etc.

Similar to medicines, exercise can also help you alleviate the symptoms of ADHD if you continue doing them. Here are some tips by which you can stay on course if you have difficulty with your attention span:

- **Move in the morning** – Try exercising first thing in the morning if it fits in your schedule. Doing it in the morning before you have taken your medications can help you get the most benefits from all the medications that you are going to take throughout the day to boost your mood. It can also help set the right tone for the rest of the day.

- **Find a partner** – Exercising with a workout buddy can help pass the time and help you stay on track while you sweat.

- **Keep it interesting** – Mix different types of exercises in your routine. If you change your activity every week or every day, it can help you stay out of a rut.

Just like any medications, the effects of exercise can only last for a specific time. Consider your workout routine as a dose of treatment. Try to exercise for thirty to forty minutes at least once a day, for four to five days a week. It is up to you to choose the kind of exercise you want to do but make sure that it is moderately intense so that your muscles feel tired, you sweat, you breathe harder and faster, and your heart rate goes up during the workout session. If you are not sure about how intense your routine should be, you should always consult your doctor. Your doctor might suggest you wear some device like a heart monitor to ensure that you are getting the most out of exercising.

Chapter 4: How Can You Minimize the Triggers?

There are so many things that can trigger your ADHD symptoms. These factors can be either environmental or biological. It differs from person to person. In this chapter, I am going to walk you through the different triggers of ADHD and what steps you can take in order to prevent them from triggering you. As you already know that ADHD is a lifelong problem, it cannot be cured. But you can definitely take steps to make the symptoms bearable, and one such step is to know your triggers and minimize them.

Some Common Triggers to be Aware of

Here is a list of common triggers responsible for making the symptoms of ADHD worse.

Food Additives

There are some parties who believe that symptoms of ADHD can be caused by additives in food, whereas there are some who oppose this view. So, a debate has been going on for quite some time. There was a review that was done in the year 2012 regarding ADHD symptoms and artificial food colorings (L. Eugene Arnold, 2012). In this review, a link was established between the two. It also stated that artificial food coloring is definitely not one of the main causes of ADHD, but it can also be said that the presence of these in food can make a child more prone to be diagnosed with ADHD. But the evidence was inconclusive, and thus, nothing can be said with certainty.

In the same year, another meta-analysis was done, and a very similar conclusion was reached to establish a link between ADHD and artificial food colorings (Joel T. Nigg, 2012). There were a total of twenty-four studies conducted under this analysis, and it said that exposure to artificial food colorings made approximately 8% of kids display ADHD symptoms.

Mineral Deficiencies

Yes, you have heard me right. Mineral deficiencies can, in fact, trigger the symptoms of ADHD. When you are under the treatment process, the medications often have a common side effect, that is, suppressed appetite (Amelia Villagomez, 2014). Stimulants mostly cause this. So, when a person is not hungry, they eat less food, and this causes several deficiencies in the body of the person, including mineral deficiencies. This can make the symptoms spiral out of control.

There are certain minerals whose deficiency in the body can cause symptoms that are very similar to that of ADHD. One such mineral is zinc, and this has been proven by research (Michael H. Bloch, 2014). The symptoms that occur as a result of zinc deficiency are the late development of cognition, restlessness, and inattentiveness.

However, I must say that there has been no conclusive study in this field that could prove that ADHD can be caused by mineral deficiencies. At the same time, levels of zinc being lower than normal has been found in children who have been diagnosed with ADHD. And these studies have also shown that using supplements of zinc during the treatment of ADHD can actually help in managing the symptoms.

Stress

Many people are confused as to whether stress can lead to ADHD in adults. Well, the ADHD episodes can definitely be triggered when you are under a lot of stress. But at the same time, you have to remember that those who have ADHD are often under a continuous state of tension and stress because their life seems to be a mess. So, it often is a vicious cycle. A person with ADHD cannot restrain from reacting severely to nominal situations, and this often leads to elevated stress levels. Other things that can add to this increasing level of stress are procrastinating about important tasks, deadlines that are knocking on the door, and not being able to focus. All of these things make the person anxious, which is, in turn, just the symptom that manifests gives rise to stress.

But we all know that stress is somewhat inevitable in our lives and so what we have to do is that we have to find a middle ground. Both emotional and cognitive challenges have to be addressed. Maintaining proper routines also helps. In Chapter 3, we already saw how mindfulness meditation could be beneficial for

ADHD, and practicing it can also help you alleviate stress.

If stress is left unmanaged, then the symptoms of ADHD can get aggravated. So, make it a practice to evaluate your stress from time to time. Follow techniques that will help you cope with your stress. I will mention some points in the second part of this chapter.

Poor Sleep

Not getting enough sleep is another of the reasons behind the symptoms of ADHD getting aggravated. Now, one of the major medications that are used for treating ADHD are stimulants, and according to the experts, these medications have the ability to cause a rise in the dopamine levels in some parts of the CNS or central nervous system and the brain. This increase in the level of dopamine is what assists in dealing with ADHD, but at the same time, it also increases the possibility of disturbed sleep or no sleep at all.

When stimulants are prescribed, a tendency of not being able to sleep is noticed in patients. In fact, they can also experience daytime sleepiness resulting from waking up from time to time at night. And, when people do not sleep well, they often feel lethargic during the day, and this, in turn, can intensify the symptoms of ADHD. It can lead to impulsivity, indecisiveness, and inattentiveness. Having a good night's sleep is very important for ADHD patients. It has also been noticed that patients often experience sleep problems when the stimulants are administered before bedtime. So, you must talk to your doctor regarding this and fix a time other than bedtime to take your medication.

You cannot afford to compromise on your sleep because it will lead to a lot of problems in your life and hamper your professional life as well. Your ability to comprehend and concentrate will decline. So, it is essential that you sleep for at least seven to eight hours every day.

Technology

There are many controversies regarding whether technology can add to the problem of ADHD and intensify the symptoms or not. It is said that symptoms can be aggravated if a person with ADHD has too much exposure to cell phones, computers, or the internet, in general. As far as watching the television is concerned, there has been confusion, but it is agreed that the symptoms are intensified to some extent. But don't get me wrong – I am not saying that loud music or watching something on the television would lead to ADHD. But if you are someone who is already struggling with increasing your concentration power, then watching television for long is only going to make it worse.

If there is some pent-up energy inside of you that you need to let go, then go and hit the gym or do some physical work. It will help you way more than just sitting in front of the TV. You can also go out with your friends and have some fun. If you are still finding it hard to regulate your time spent in front of the TV, then I would say that you should form a routine where you will have fixed hours throughout the day for everything. This will help you set limited time frames for watching TV or anything that involves you sitting in front of the screen. In fact, there have been several studies that say computer screens, televisions, and mobile phones can cause overstimulation that triggers ADHD symptoms.

Even though there are no specific formal guidelines that tell you the number of hours that can be spent in front of the screen for an ADHD patient, but you can try limiting it after consulting with your doctor.

Tips for Minimizing Triggers

So, now that you know about the common triggers of ADHD symptoms, here are some tips on how you can reduce them.

Maintain a Balanced Diet

Maintaining a balanced diet is very important for not only reducing the triggers but also for preventing ADHD, according to some studies. But what is a balanced diet? Well, a simple definition of a balanced diet is something that includes a well-proportionate amount of all nutrients. So, the foods that you should definitely include in your diet are whole grains, whole fruits, vegetables, different protein sources, healthy fats (oils like olive oil, canola oil, and so on), low-fat dairy, and so on. If you are not aware of where to start then, you can consult a dietician.

If you are taking stimulant medications for ADHD, then you might face symptoms of appetite suppression, and it is quite common. So, you have to make sure that your diet has all the important nutrients; otherwise, you will become deficient in several essential nutrients. If you see that your weight is reducing drastically, then you should consult your doctor because your medication might need to be changed. You might be given an alternate medicine, or your dosage might be adjusted.

Exercise Regularly

I have already emphasized the importance of exercise in Chapter 3. You will also find some common exercises to start with in that chapter. It has been noticed that regular exercise in ADHD patients has helped them improve their cognitive performance to some extent.

Apart from exercise, you should also try mindfulness meditation because it will help you calm your mind and also relieve yourself from stress.

Work On Your Time Management Skills

It is important for every adult suffering from ADHD to brush up on their time management skills. Missing deadlines and procrastinating are very common in patients with ADHD, and this is also what leads to stress. The idea of time is very differently perceived in patients with ADHD as compared to others and so, working on time management skills is so important. It is important that you keep a clock on your desk at all times, which will help you keep track of time. Moreover, take note of the time when you are starting your task and then plant to finish it within a certain time period. For this, you can use timers. Working within a limited time span will prevent the ADHD mind from being scattered and inattentive. The timer will let you know when your limited time is over. If you are doing something that required you to work for an extended period of time, then you can set your timer to go off after regular intervals. After each interval, you can take five-minute breaks. This will help in boosting your productivity. Maintaining a timer like this will also keep you aware of the amount of time that is passing by.

It is also important to make the right estimation of the time that you are going to need. Don't constrict your tasks within a very short span of time. This will put too much stress on you. So, even if you think you are going to need an hour for a task, make sure you keep ten minutes extra on top of the one hour so that you have a time cushion.

In the same way, if you have an appointment at 5 pm, note it down in your calendar at 4:50 pm so that you have ten minutes extra at hand. This will give you time to prepare or have your back even if you are late for some reason. You should set reminders for even the smallest task so that you don't forget anything.

Spend Time Outdoors

Even if you are not exercising or going for a morning run, it is important that you spend some of your time outdoors in nature. Working out is, of course, the best option. But if you don't feel like it on some days, just go to the park and sit on a bench. The sunshine and the fresh air is going to help a lot in reducing stress. Try to spend time somewhere where there is lush greenery. If you live in a city, go to a park. The greenery is soothing to the eyes and has a feel-good vibe.

Get Enough Sleep

Like I told you before, ADHD symptoms can get triggered when you are not getting proper sleep. So, if you want to stay attentive during the day and work productively, then you need to sleep properly at night. The first thing that you need to do is not having caffeine in the second half of the day. Exercising regularly also helps in having a good sleep but make sure you don't exercise just before going to bed. Your sleeping cycle has to be maintained even on weekends. Maintain a fixed time not only for waking up in the morning but also for going to bed at night. This will bring you into a fixed routine and will help your body adjust to its sleep-wake cycle. Create your own bedtime routine that is not too elaborate and yet gives you peace. It can be taking a soothing bath and then using some relaxing skin products. You can listen to a particular soothing playlist or whatever makes you feel relaxed.

For some people, drinking a cup of warm tea is helpful. But you should select the right tea as well. Chamomile tea is really great for sleep. Whatever tea you choose, you need to make sure that there is no caffeine content in it. Make your dinner light. If your dinner is too heavy, you are more likely to feel bloated. This causes discomfort and hampers sleep. So, you can even have a light snack.

Before going to bed, you need to prepare your brain for sleep. So, you can practice some quiet time. This means that you have to practice relaxation and not listen to anything loud or watch TV. You can even practice reading a bit if that is something you love to do. You can play sounds of ocean waves or crickets because they are highly relaxing.

Some ADHD patients have also said that aromatherapy has helped them a lot in terms of sleeping. So, you can try oils like chamomile, jasmine, and lavender because all of them are well known for promoting good sleep.

Try to think about happy things before going to bed. Steer clear of all those negative thoughts because they are not going to help you in any way. Practicing positive thinking is really a good habit to release stress and prevent anxiety during bedtime.

You need to avoid all those things that can hamper your sleep. This also includes sugary foods. When you eat or drinks sugary items, it automatically gives your body an energy boost, which is also known as the sugar rush. It keeps you awake and is, thus, not ideal before bedtime.

While you can practice these strategies on your own, if you think that you are being triggered frequently, it is best that you consult with your doctor.

Chapter 5: Behavioral Therapy for ADHD

It is the medication that helps an ADHD patient on the neurological level, but in order to make day-to-day life easier, therapy is extremely important. Behavioral therapy is a basic or preliminary therapeutic approach that an ADHD patient is exposed to. The therapy starts in their childhood years. In adulthood, the therapy changes into CBT or Cognitive Behavioral Therapy. Before moving into the details of CBT, I would like to briefly discuss with you the behavioral therapy in kids.

How Does Behavioral Therapy Work?

When we talk about going to therapy, what we picture in our minds is a therapist talking to his/her patient. But that is not how every type of therapy looks like. In fact, behavioral therapy is quite different. Here, the emotions of the person are not the main focus – the focus is on the actions and how they can be rectified.

When a child or an adult is taken to a therapist, the therapist will first understand the state of the problem and then prepare a plan with the help of which you can work towards solving your problem. The main idea is to get rid of all the toxic and negative habits and simultaneously, replacing those bad things with positive habits. In the case of kids, behavioral therapy does not only involve the kids but also the parents.

This is because the parents are the ones responsible for the upbringing of the child – they have a great influence on the mind of the child. There are so many parents of ADHD kids who get frustrated and start yelling at the kid even though the kid did not do it on purpose. So, a major part of behavioral therapy is also about making parents understand their kids and change their own behaviors towards the kids.

No matter what the type of behavioral therapy is, a system of rewards and consequences is always set up. The rewards have to be chosen very carefully. The rewards have to be something that motivates the patient and makes him/her truly work hard towards achieving their goals.

There are a lot of ways in which behavioral therapy can be helpful. In the case of kids, it helps them in keeping their anger in check and then slowly helps themselves get adjusted to social settings. They learn how they should perceive each situation and then react in a reasonable manner. They learn various tactics of self-control. Since the main aim is to inculcate good habits in the child, the rewards that are chosen for the therapy should also reinforce good behavior in the patient.

But when you notice that rewards are not really helpful, then you have to take a different approach. That is when the concept of consequences, particularly negative consequences, walks in. If the patient does not do something as asked, then he/she will lose points – this is what negative consequences look like.

CBT for Adults

There have several research and clinical results that support the fact that adults with ADHD can benefit a lot from CBT or cognitive behavioral therapy. The patient is not only happier, but they also show higher levels of happiness, are highly productive, and their self-esteem also gets a boost. Here, in this section, I am going to tell you more about CBT and how it helps ADHD patients.

What Is CBT?

Cognitive behavioral therapy or CBT is primarily a talking therapy, and it is done over the short-term to bring a change in the way people think and instill healthy thought patterns. Adults with ADHD have already undergone a lifetime of poor self-esteem, continually missing deadlines, and forgetfulness. But this goal-oriented therapy that mostly involves concepts of psychotherapy can help the patient change his/her thoughts about the world, their own self, and their future. All the negative thoughts are replaced with positive ones. In short, CBT can be termed as specialized training for the brain.
The main idea behind CBT is to bring a change in how the person perceives the events of their lives. It also deals with how they behave in such situations. Both these things ultimately have an immense effect on how the person feels. Whether a person is dealing

with complicated relationships, stress, or negativity, CBT can help in every aspect. In fact, studies have proven the usefulness of CBT. The quality of life of the patient can be significantly improved by introducing CBT. This therapy is not only used in the case of ADHD patients but for a whole range of other problems as well. These include drug use problems, alcohol problems, anxiety problems, and also depression. It has also been noticed that compared to other forms of psychiatric medications, CBT can give better results.

The main principles on which the idea of CBT is based are as follows –

- It is considered that partly, every psychological problem is somehow a result of unhelpful or faulty thinking patterns.

- It is also considered that partly, every psychological problem is a result of unhelpful or learned behavioral patterns.

- Better coping methods can be learned by patients with a psychological problem, which would help them manage their symptoms and lead a better life.

So, if we have to put in words, CBT is not only a goal-oriented treatment method but also one that is very specific to the problem at hand. It addresses the behaviors and thoughts of the patient and all the challenges they are facing in the present day. CBT can be done in both group and one-on-one therapy sessions. So, honestly, it is quite a broad concept, and the treatment can be designed to focus on specific aspects of your life. But both the counselor and the patient will have to collaborate together in order to make it work. There will be a series of sessions.

Initially, CBT was mainly used for people suffering from mood disorders. After that, it branched out to other problems. All of us have automatic thoughts as a reaction to different situations. But these thoughts are the reason why we face so many problems in our emotional state. CBT addresses these thoughts and helps you correct your spontaneous interpretation of things. Our spontaneous interpretations are not always correct, and the main reason behind this is that they are biased and influenced by different types of distortions. These internal dialogs are so ingrained in our minds that they act as an obstruction in making the right decision. So, whenever you are trying to calculate the risk or do something productive, your mental distortions will hinder you.

But once you start CBT, you will notice what a significant impact it can have on your life. Completing tasks and staying on a particular task for an extended period will become easier with CBT because the problematic thought patterns will be changed. All the distorted cognitions that you have will be challenged by CBT, and thus, your behavioral patterns will change.

How Does CBT Help ADHD Adults?

Now, let us see how CBT works to give you a better life. As you already know, the self-regulation skills of people are gravely affected through ADHD. The direct result of this is that the executive functioning skills of the adult are affected. It is also why ADHD adults suffer from emotional dysregulation, disastrous time management skills, inconsistent motivation, disorganization, procrastination, and impulsivity. But all these problems that I have mentioned here are not yet included in the different criteria for diagnosing ADHD even though the patients display these symptoms.

It is often seen that adults who have been diagnosed with ADHD have a pessimistic attitude towards life. They become highly self-critical. The main reason behind all of this is that there are several setbacks that they have to endure both in everyday life and social settings. When situations don't go as planned (which is often the case), ADHD patients spiral into a cycle of self-blame. But what is worse is that these patients start projecting their pessimistic thoughts onto their future as well. Just because they had a bad day, they think that every other day that is going to come will be bad as well.

ADHD patients can't seem the logic in things because their thought processes are entirely clouded by their demoralizing beliefs and thoughts. It also hinders their possibility of growth and being productive.

Here, I am going to list of the distorted thinking patterns that adults with ADHD experience. CBT helps in correcting all these patterns –

- **All-or-nothing thinking** – This type of thinking pattern is when a person consistently uses words like ever or never (i.e., absolute words). This thinking pattern is very common in people irrespective of whether they have ADHD or not. When someone indulges in this type of thinking, they can only think in extremes. No matter how much they try, they cannot seem to get out of the black-and-white terms. What they have to do is understand that there are a lot of gray areas in life. This faulty thinking pattern also makes people overlook any alternative solutions that might be present. And in the case of ADHD patients, this type of thinking promotes them to think only about the downside of things. Thus, these patients either see themselves as a complete failure, or they think they are highly successful. If they make a small mistake in their project, they immediately start discrediting all of the efforts they have put into the project and start thinking that they have failed.

- **Mind reading** – This cognitive distortion is when a person automatically assumes that they know what the person in front of them is thinking. This distortion is very dangerous because people fail to notice what is right in front of them just because they are too engrossed in their idea of things. They rely so much on their self-proclaimed ability to read minds that they sometimes end up misreading others' intentions. It leads to sudden bouts of frustration and anxiety. The direct result of mind reading is social anxiety, and in the case of ADHD patients, this is even more magnified because ADHD adults already suffer from a certain extent of social anxiety.

- **Overgeneralization** – Overgeneralization is when people make some pretty broad assumptions about things even when their experience in that matter is limited. There are different forms in which overgeneralization can manifest itself. But it mostly revolves around the fact that once a person notices something negative, they start thinking everything is going to be negative. In short, they allow one singular event to predict every outcome that is to follow. For example, just because you didn't get the job after giving an interview, you start thinking you are not going to get any of them because you are not good enough. This thought process brings about a feeling of hopelessness.

- **Fortune-telling** – This is another type of cognitive distortion seen in ADHD patients where they claim that they know the future, and it is going to be bad. The roots of this type of thought pattern are based on anxiety. But there is a difference between making an educated guess and fortune-telling. When you are predicting things simply on the basis of assumptions, that is when you are fortune-telling as a part of your cognitive distortion. Thus, the real odds are never considered, and so you cannot call fortune telling a real form of assessment. For example, if your job interview went bad, you can probably assess it, but there is no way of knowing for sure whether or not you are going to get the job. There might be a hundred reasons why you will get the job. You don't know how your competitors performed or whether their personality is a good fit for the job. So, if you still assume that you are not going to get the job despite the fact that you don't know a lot of factors, then you are fortune-telling.

- **Personalization** – This is another type of cognitive distortion that ADHD adults go through. In this type of negative thought pattern, the person keeps blaming themselves for everything that happened wrong. Or, the person blames someone else. No matter who the person is blaming, the situation was totally out of control, and in reality, no one is at fault. For example, when ADHD patients cannot perform well in a professional career, they blame themselves that only if they had put in some more effort, there would have been no complications. But things are not like that –

ADHD is a problem whose symptoms will hamper your everyday life, and you have no control over that.

- **Comparative thinking** – This type of thinking is what brings inferiority complexes and makes us feel that we cannot achieve things. Sometimes, the comparisons made are not even realistic, and yet people continue to believe them. ADHD patients have been commonly found to give in to comparative thinking. Every person on earth has his/her own weaknesses and strengths, and so comparisons are not something that you should do.

- **Mental filtering** – This is a specific type of faulty thought pattern that is found not only in people with ADHD but also in others. When a person has the habit of mental filtering, he/she filters out all the good and positive things and directs all their focus on the negative things. Thus, in simpler terms, people with mental filtering are the ones who always find their glass half empty. They are so focused on their dissatisfaction and inadequacies that they miss out on all the fun. Their feels are often rooted in loneliness. The only way to overcome this particular cognitive distortion is to focus on reframing your negative thoughts.

- **Emotional reasoning** – Lastly, this is another type of cognitive distortion commonly seen in ADHD patients where they think that their reality is reflected by their negative feelings. So, let us say that you are tensed, and so you think you are in danger – this is what emotional reasoning looks like. This often leads to exaggerations of problems that are too insignificant.

When you go for CBT, your therapist will help you understand your thoughts, and you will also learn to identify the different types of cognitive distortions on your own. When you widen your perception of a situation, your reaction is also expanded into something that is less defensive. With CBT, you will learn to address your fears and your insecurities slowly but steadily. There will be plenty of activities through which the therapist will ease you into the process. There will be role-playing activities and also assignments given to you as a part of your homework.

With time, you will notice that you no longer jump to conclusions like before, or you don't give in to a negative mindset as your default setting. One very common problem among patients of ADHD is procrastination. Keeping track of time seems to be a major issue, but not everyone suffers in the same way. For each patient, the therapist will ask him/her to describe a recent situation where procrastination got the better of them. After listening to the incident, a specific goal for that patient will be set. The goal can be something as commonplace as shopping groceries.

The relationship of the patient with that of the task is analyzed because this will help the therapist chalk out the plan that you are going to follow. After that, the task will be broken down into simple, actionable steps. Each step is then analyzed to find out whether any potential barriers might arise and if yes, then what steps can be followed to overcome those barriers. While doing all of this, the therapist will also ask the patient about what they are thinking during each step. They will also you what emotions are crossing your mind and how do you feel when you are finally facing the task that you had been putting off for so long.

I am not saying that the process is going to be easy because it won't. There will be a lot of obstacles that you will have to cross in order to be successful. But what is invaluable is the fact that you will be discussing your ADHD problems at length with a professional, and this itself is going to be so refreshing and helpful. In fact, some patients also say that the mere act of discussion is so therapeutic.

You should also keep in mind that in order to get success through CBT, you also need to go to an expert. Also, since CBT is used for a variety of psychological problems, there are several CBT therapists who are not aware of how to treat ADHD. So, whoever you got to just make sure you have asked them about their experience of handling ADHD patients. The ADHD specialty clinics are now growing in number with each passing day, and you can also contact these clinics to know about any qualified therapists near you who can help you with CBT. So, if an orderly life is what you want, don't waste any more time and look for a CBT specialist today.

Another thing for which you will get help from CBT is the comorbid conditions. Hypersensitivity often leads to anxiety, and CBT helps address all the issues and comorbid conditions of ADHD. Every condition is treated with a different approach in the case of CBT.

What Is DBT?

Next up, we are going to discuss another type of therapy option that is available for ADHD adults, and it is known as Dialectical Behavioral Therapy. It is quite similar to CBT because this one is also focused on mitigating the challenges faced by a patient on an emotional and social level.

Initially, it was only the patients of BPD or borderline personality who were treated with DBT, but now, it is being used in several problems. The therapy mainly focuses on teaching emotional regulation skills, and in the case of ADHD patients, these skills prove to be very fruitful in leading an everyday life.

Chapter 6: A Step-by-Step Guide to Become More Productive With ADHD

Adults with ADHD often go through days when they feel like they cannot do anything. They cannot think straight, nor can they stay focused on any task—this inability to focus hampers their productivity levels. But the worst part is that this feeling is very often what every day looks like for an ADHD patient. We all know that when it comes to productivity, the most common rules that apply to usual circumstances are prioritize, focus, and delegate. However, these rules cannot be used in the case of an ADHD patient. It is because the ADHD brain works differently.

But no matter how many obstacles stand in your path, it doesn't mean that you cannot be productive. You can definitely learn some strategies that will help you manage your time and stay up to date with work. So, in this chapter, we are going to have a look at some of the most common productivity tips that are extremely useful for ADHD patients and will help you handle every distraction that comes your way.

Step 1 - Don't Try Multitasking

People often think that multitasking is the answer to your problems but trust me, it is not. Multitasking will only complicate things further for an ADHD patient.

If you want to get something done, the first and foremost thing is that you need to stay focused. So, for a person who is easily distracted, doing one thing at a time is a big challenge. If that person were to do multiple things at a time, think how hard it is going to be for him/her to stay focused. Every task on that person's list ends up staying incomplete.

You might think that multitasking is going to save time, but it is quite the opposite. When you have to do many things at once, the ADHD brain is not able to work efficiently. The main reason behind this is that there is a constant shift of focus from one task to another, so the brain basically keeps doing back and forth. Every time the brain has to focus on something new, it takes a couple of seconds to readjust. Even if it doesn't seem much to you, these seconds keep adding up, and at the end of the day, multitasking is the reason why you are left with incomplete tasks.

But the problem is, multitasking has become like second nature to most of us. Here are some things that you can do to avoid multitasking –

- Firstly, you have to find out the pairs of activities that you usually tend to multitask. Then, sort them into groups. All tasks that have some kind of familiarity between them can be sorted together in one group. For example, you can watch TV and file your nails at the same time. But you definitely should not answer your emails while watching TV. The idea is to separate the daily tasks which can be grouped together to multitask and save time. But the more complex tasks should be set aside.

- For the tasks that you have pointed out as complex, you need to block time in your planner. This time span will be solely devoted to completing that one single task. When you are spending time doing that one single task, you need to keep your phone away. You can also put up a board on your door that says 'do not disturb.' If you think that the new project that has been assigned to you is not the typical easy ones and you need extra time to complete it, then let your client know about it.

- Try developing a morning routine. A morning routine might not be directly related to multitasking, but it helps you establish a pattern, and you will do the same things every day in the same order. Moreover, a routine will increase your familiarity with a single task, and the more you do it, the more familiar you will find it. And then, after a certain point of time, that task might become so familiar to you that you can add it to your list of tasks that are multitaskable.

Lastly, I would like to say, no matter what, you should try not to multitask because it has been seen that the more people try to multitask, the more they are late at completing things. This makes them work on the weekends or stay up late every night just to catch up with everything. The result of all this is stress, and you definitely don't want more of that in your life.

Step 2 - Be Realistic

Being realistic is one of the major things to learn in order to increase your productivity with ADHD. You have to understand that since you have ADHD, your brain is not like that of others. It is different, and the concept of time is also different.

So, when you decide a time frame for your tasks, you need to be quite realistic about it. Keep in mind that every task is going to take much longer than you think it would. So, plan some extra time in your schedules so that you don't have to run at the last minute to cover your deadline. Also, whenever you are planning your tasks and your time frames, include small breaks in between. This will prevent your brain from getting tired, and you will stay energized throughout. Taking breaks in between is all the more important for patients with ADHD; otherwise, your concentration levels will falter.

Thus, you simply have to follow the rule of 'under-promise and over-deliver.' Make it your motto. If you are an optimistic and career-oriented person, you already have an idea in your mind regarding the number of things you can do in a day. But when you promise people around you that you are going to deliver the service within a time period and then fail to deliver it, there is no value in your promise. Moreover, this will also create a constant pressure upon you. So, the trick is to commit less and deliver more. This will not only enhance the satisfaction of the clients but also improve your productivity levels and give you more motivation.

Step 3 – Stop Trying to be Perfect

The need to be perfect at all times is often the biggest hindrance that we have on our paths. And for an ADHD patient, this is all the more true. You have to understand that sometimes it is okay to make mistakes and not do things perfectly. In order to be productive, sometimes you have to allow your laundry to keep stacking in the corner of the room and order takeout. You need to learn to cut yourself some slack from time to time because you are not a machine. Perfectionism is your enemy, and you cannot give in to it. The more you chase perfectionism, the more you will ask yourself whether you are enough. The truth is – 'You are enough.' It doesn't require you to be perfect to be enough. Being perfect is an illusion, and you have to break free.

If you think that you want to be perfect, then you will constantly be chasing something or the other in your life – be it more beauty, wealth, more promotions, or anything. The road of being perfect is always dissatisfying because it will drive you down a track where you will keep wanting for more, and there is no end to that.

Don't depend on others to make you feel worthy because that is also how perfectionism keeps growing. You will never feel enough if you keep relying on others. It is a deceptive cycle. External validation will inevitably make you feel that you need more to feel enough. So, you need to bring a change to your mindset. Set expectations that are realistic and always put your well-being first. Your perception of the world depends quite largely on how you see it. People are not born with the idea of self-reliance. You have to learn it. The moment you do that, you will realize that you are in more control of the situation than you thought you were. It will not only boost your happiness but also your sense of self-esteem. Accept yourself for the person you are.

Stop telling yourself that you are a failure. This type of negative self-talk is not going to get you anywhere in life. It will not convince you to accept yourself. What you need to do is make yourself believe that you are good just the way you are.

One of the most prominent aspects of striving to be perfect is the need to always get it right. The moment things go a bit off-road, people feel like a failure. But you have to make yourself understand that the fact that you are trying to achieve your goal and putting yourself out there is a huge accomplishment. So, make progress and give a pat on your back because you deserve it.

Step 4 – Prep Your Environment

The next thing to do if you want to be productive is to prep your environment. It will elevate productivity levels by helping you to focus. Whether you are working from home or from your office, your environment plays a significant role in your productivity.

Here are some things that you should keep in mind –

- **Lighting** – The first aspect to take care of is the lighting. If you want to feel inspired to work and churn out more ideas, you'd be amazed to know what a great role lighting plays in it. But even then, people often overlook this factor. You will feel irritated and put a lot of strain on your eyes when your workspace doesn't have sufficient lighting. In fact, it has been found that people become depressed when they work in dark spaces. If you are working from your cubicle at the office and the general lighting is not enough, don't be shy to bring your own light. But if you are working from home, things are in your control. So, allow as much natural light as you can. Open all the windows. If the day is cloudy, make sure you switch on the lights.

- **Table and chair** – Now, let us talk about the type of chair and table that you should use. When your table and chair are not of the right type, you will often find yourself moving or stretching from time to time. For the best ergonomics, your feet should not be dangling. They should be either resting on the floor or on a footrest. Your eye level should match with that of the top of the monitor. The distance between your eyes and the computer screen should be at least 24-36 inches. In order to avoid or prevent any kind of back pain, the chair posture needs to be a bit reclined. But if you are working in a company, you can't do anything about the chair. What you can do is add some pillows to adjust your back. But if you are having a height problem with the chair, you can ask for a riser. Investing in a good-quality chair is what you should do if you are working from your home.

- **Reduce clutter** — ADHD patients often forget to clean their spaces, but clutter will only hamper your productivity, and you cannot afford to do that. In your office, you obviously do not have control over the clutter generated in the whole area. But you can definitely keep your own workspace clean. Make it a routine to clean your desk every evening before you leave, and every morning when you come. Just set everything in place and start your day fresh. It will help minimize the distraction. When you are working from home, the chances of clutter increase a lot. Everything that is in your house can distract you. If you are someone who stays busy most of the time, then you will need to have a professional cleaner to help you out. But if you want to save money, then you have to fix a day in a week when you will clean everything. Apart from this, set aside fifteen minutes of your time every day to clean your home office.

- **Room temperature** – You might be surprised to know that room temperature does play a role in your productivity. It applies even more to ADHD patients because they tend to get irritated by the slightest things. Your productivity increases with warmer rooms. But in offices, the general temperature that is maintained is 65-68 F, and this is not the ideal range for productivity. Since you cannot control the temperature of your office, you can bring a space heater for your cabin. But if you are at home, you need to adjust the temperature depending on the weather.

- **Room scents** – Your mood is hugely affected by the different scents in your surroundings, and so you should do something about it. If you feel that you have been drifting off quite frequently, then keeping some aromatic substances in your surroundings might help you focus. For example, the smell of cinnamon can help you maintain your focus for longer periods, the smell of citrus helps in lifting up your mood and keeps you awake, the smell of lavender should be used after a long and tiring day at work to help you relax, and the smell of pine keeps you alert. Remember that if you are working in an area where you have others close to you, then you should use scents that are subtle and won't disturb others. But if you are at home, then you can use essential oils or candles.

- **Level of noise** – The level of noise is something that is very often not in our hands to control. The company culture and the size of your team are some of the things affecting the noise. The design of your office also plays a role. But we cannot deny the fact that our concentration levels depend on the noise to a huge extent. If the levels are way above average, then you might find it difficult to concentrate, and your productivity will take a hit. While working from home, people often think that maintaining a quiet space can be attention boosting, but it is quite the opposite. Complete silence is often a distraction in itself. So, you can play some mild sounds that boost your concentration. White noise is a very good example. If you are working from your office or a place that is too noisy, always carry your noise-canceling headphones. They can be a real savior in such situations.

Step 5 – Time Your Tasks

In this step, we are going to learn how you can time your tasks and how beneficial it is when it comes to time management. Timing your tasks can actually give you a better sense of time. And it is also quite simple to do. All you need is to set the alarm on your phone or use a timer. ADHD patients often struggle with procrastination. Timing the tasks will help you deal with it effectively. Fix a particular amount of time for a particular task and then start working. But whatever time you choose, make sure you are not pushing yourself too much. You will know that it is time to start the next task when your timer goes off.

Similarly, when ADHD patients start doing something that they love, they tend to spend the entire day on the task. In order to prevent that, timing the task will let you know that you have already spent a specific amount of time on that task, and now, it is time to move on. It is advisable that you use a timer for every task that you do in the day, be it running errands for home or working on projects at your office.

Timing your tasks will also help you keep track of all those areas where you are less productive, and then, you can work on these areas separately. Every activity that is present on your to-do list for the day should be assigned a specific time span.

Step 6 – Do the Fun Stuff First

I know that many of you believe in doing the difficult things first so that by the time half the day has passed, you are done with the tricky tasks. But in the case of ADHD patients, if the day starts with tasks that pose a lot of resistance, it is easier for them to lose focus. So, it is advised that you do the easier things first. Or, you can start with the things you love doing.

Moreover, when you finish the good things first, it will not take you much time. The sense of accomplishment that you will get on completing those tasks will motivate you to work more and get more things done.

Taking small steps at the beginning of the day will prevent you from getting overwhelmed.

Step 7 – Use Visual Reminders

Visual reminders have often proved to be very helpful for ADHD patients to remember stuff. Moreover, you can be as creative as you want while planning these visual reminders. Decorate your office walls with boards where you can put up your deadlines and personal acronyms to remind you of the tasks that you need to get done. You can also put up rules that you need to follow.

Make sure you put up these reminders and deadlines where it is easy for you to notice them. It will also constantly remind you to use your time productively. You can also take the help of sticky notes to put up reminders on your desk, on your computer screen, or wherever you feel would be easier to notice. You can also set productive screensavers on your computer so that even when you are taking a break, you always have a quote boosting you up.

So, I hope that you follow all these steps mentions here, but the most important thing to keep in mind is that our own negative self-talk is what holds us back. No matter how many tips you follow, if you don't stop automatic negation in your mind, it is only going to put you in a counterproductive path.

Chapter 7: Treating ADHD With Medication

Is it okay to use medications for ADHD? Do these medications have any side effects? I understand that you might have several such questions in your mind, and in this chapter, we are going to address all those issues.

It is true that the symptoms of ADHD can be kept in control with the help of medication. This applies to both adults and children. You can get a hold on impulsivity, inattentiveness, and hyperactivity by taking the right medications. But you also have to understand that there are several risks and side effects associated with these medications. Moreover, if you have gone through Chapter 5, then you already know that medications are not the only form of treatment option available to you. Whether you are an ADHD patient yourself or a family member, it is of utmost importance that you have all the knowledge about ADHD medications. Having a comprehensive knowledge will help you make the right decisions and go with the best options.

Before going into too many details, one of the most basic things to understand is how these medications can help an ADHD patient and what their limitations are. For starters, taking the right medications will help the patient stay focused on the task at hand, plan things properly, and get a grip on their impulses. But you also have to remember that medications cannot do any magic. You will notice that the patient is suffering from certain symptoms like social anxiety and forgetfulness from time to time, even when they are taking the medications. So, a lot of other changes in the daily lifestyle of the patient is also required for any long-term change. This includes maintaining a proper sleep cycle, following a healthy diet, and doing some regular exercise.

Remember that no matter what medication you use, ADHD is a lifelong problem, and it will not be cured by medication. But when you take the meds, you will get relief from the nagging symptoms. Some patients think that now that they are not having symptoms, they can stop the meds. But the moment they do that, the symptoms come back, and they are worse. Another thing to keep in mind is that the medications don't work equally on everyone. If someone you know is benefitting a lot from a certain medication, it is not that you will get the same level of benefits. You might only notice some modest development while the other person might witness dramatic changes. The reaction of a patient to a particular ADHD medication is quite unpredictable. The main reason behind this is that every person has a different response to the medication.

That is why when you visit a doctor, he/she will diagnose you, examine the intensity and type of your symptoms, and then prescribe you a dosage that is solely meant for you. The medications are extremely personalized. Even after that, you should visit the doctor for regular check-ups. ADHD might go out of hand and become a risk if you do not visit the doctor from time to time. The medications need to be monitored very closely.

Stimulant Medications

There are basically two groups of medications that are used in the treatment process of this disorder. One of them is the stimulant medications. They mostly help you by controlling hyperactivity, reigning in impulsive behavior, and stretching the short attention span of the patient. Sometimes, patients are treated solely with the help of stimulant medication, and at other times, some kind of therapy is used along with the meds.

It has been found that about 70-80% of the children and 70% of the adults with ADHD have seen an improvement in their symptoms once they started using stimulant medications. The meds have also proved to be fruitful in helping patients to improve their relationships. If the patients keep on taking the medications without fail, then they witness not only better behavioral tendencies but also a much more focused life. However, there is still not enough evidence supporting the fact that medications can help in regulating the social life of patients.

Another interesting fact to keep in mind about the stimulant medications is that they have been in use for the longest time when it comes to ADHD treatment. Their effectiveness in this field is backed up several studies. Some familiar names in this group of medications are Dexedrine, Adderall, and Ritalin.

The main working mechanism of stimulant drugs is that they help in increasing the levels of dopamine in the brain. Now, for your knowledge, there are several neurotransmitters in the brain, and dopamine is just one of them. It is mainly responsible for movement, attention, pleasure, and motivation. Most ADHD patients have reported that they have received significant benefits after taking stimulant medications in terms of improved focus and concentration levels.

Now, there are two types of stimulant medications that are used. They are as follows –

- **Long-acting stimulants** – These medications are usually prescribed to be taken only once in a day. It is because their effect lingers for a long time period, usually for about eight to twelve hours. They are also known as extended-release stimulants. These medications are also more commonly preferred. When people have ADHD, they have trouble remembering stuff, and so, if they have to take medications multiple times in a day, it becomes difficult. But in the case of long-acting stimulants, they only need to take the meds once a day. Thus, it is a much more convenient option.

- **Short-acting stimulants** – The other type of stimulant medications are the short-acting ones. As the name suggests, the effect of these meds is very short-lived, and their peak effect is felt after several hours of consumption. They need to be taken at least two times a day and sometimes even three.

Now, let us talk about some of the common side effects that stimulant medications have –

- Upset stomach
- Dizziness
- Frequent mood swings and irritability
- Feeling jittery and restless
- Tics
- Sleeping irregularities
- Headache
- Fast-paced heartbeat
- Increase in blood pressure
- Reduced appetite
- Depression
- Nervousness

Apart from the ones that are mentioned above, some patients also notice changes in their personality after taking stimulant medications. Some people have reported becoming more talkative, whereas others become rigid or listless. There have also been cases where patients became less spontaneous and somewhat withdrawn from life.

There are certain side effects that do not linger for long. These include upset stomach and headache. They might go away once the patient becomes accustomed to the medication. Your body will take time to adjust itself to this new medication, but once that time period is over, you should get better. But you will have to inform your doctor if the side effects remain for a longer time.

For side effects that don't go away on their own, a change in medication is usually required. In some cases, people are allergic to certain stimulant medications. The allergy might manifest itself in the form of a rash or skin pigmentation. Keep an eye out for such signs, and if you notice anything of that sort, you have to inform your doctor at once.

Now that we have discussed the different side effects of these medications, it is time you are made known about other safety concerns that are associated with taking stimulant medications.

- **Heart** – Let us first see what effect these medications have on your heart. When adults with pre-existing heart conditions take these stimulant medications over the long-term, sudden death has been noticed in some of these patients. That is why it is advised by experts before you start any type of stimulant medication for ADHD, you should definitely get a cardiac evaluation done. And, if the person already has a history of problems related to the cardiovascular system, then an electrocardiogram should be done.

- **Developing brain** – When stimulant medications are administered to kids with ADHD or adolescents, the effect on the developing brain has not yet been clearly determined. But it is a common fear among the researchers that brain development might be hampered when children are exposed to stimulant medications over the long-term.

- **Substance abuse** – It is a very growing concern among the families of ADHD patients because stimulant medications often lead to substance abuse problems. This is even more common in young adults and teens. The fact that stimulant medications can cause a loss in weight has also added to this problem. So, if someone in your house is taking the stimulant medication, you have to be aware as to whether they are selling these or sharing them with someone else.

- **Psychiatric problems** – Some psychiatric problems are triggered by the use of stimulant medications. These problems include paranoia, depression, anxiety, aggression, and hostility. If the ADHD patient already has a family history of bipolar disorder, depression, or suicide, then they are more at risk of developing these problems. So, when a patient is taking stimulant medications, they should miss an appointment with their doctor because these medications have to be closely monitored at all times.

Here is a list of people who are advised against taking stimulant medications –

- Patients who have been diagnosed with a coronary artery disease

- Patients who have hyperthyroidism

- Patients who already have past instances of drug abuse

- Patients who suffer from problems where their heartbeat is not normal and is irregular

- Patients who have glaucoma

- Patients who have been found to be allergic to stimulant medications

- Patients who suffer from frequent bouts of anxiety

- Patients who have had psychotic episodes in the past

- Patients with tics

If you are still confused about when you should call your doctor, then here are some red flags that you should be aware of –

- Fainting

- Difficulty in breathing

- Pain in the chest

- Paranoia or suspicion

- Having auditory or visual hallucinations

If you notice any of the above-mentioned signs in the patient, you need to call the doctor at once.

Non-Stimulant Medications

In the previous section, we talked about stimulant mediations, but they are not the only type of drugs used to control ADHD symptoms. There is another type of drug known as non-stimulant drugs. These include several medications used for controlling blood pressure, antidepressants, and also Strattera. Usually, doctors don't prescribe non-stimulant medications right away. The first choice is always the stimulant medication. But if the patient cannot be prescribed stimulant medication due to some existing health problems or the stimulant medications are not working for him/her, then the non-stimulant medications are prescribed.

So, let us talk about these non-stimulant medications one by one.

Strattera. This non-stimulant is used for ADHD treatment quite commonly, and it has also been approved by the FDA. The medicines are also popularly known by its generic name – which is – atomoxetine. In the previous section, I told you how the dopamine levels in the brain are affected by stimulant medications. In the case of Strattera, it is the levels of norepinephrine that is increased.

When compared to the other types of non-stimulant medications, it is found that the effect of Strattera on the human body is quite long-lived. In fact, you can get relief from the symptoms for an entire day. Thus, for people who find it challenging to get up in the morning, this medication is quite a good option. Another positive point about Strattera is that it helps in curbing depression. So, if a patient is already suffering from depression and anxiety along with ADHD, then Strattera is a very good choice of medication for them. Moreover, it doesn't matter whether the patient has Tourette's Syndrome or tics; they can still have this medication. Aside from all this, the effectiveness of Strattera in treating the symptoms of ADHD are comparable to that of stimulant medications.

Some of the commonly seen side effects in patients using Strattera are as follows – frequent mood swings, vomiting or nausea, upset stomach, pain in the abdomen, dizziness, headache, and feeling lethargic or sleepy. Some uncommon side effects of Strattera are reduced appetite and difficulty in sleeping.

Now, let us move on to some other types of non-stimulants that are used in the treatment of ADHD. But these are not approved by the FDA and are 'off-label.' These medications are not usually prescribed by doctors until and unless Straterra doesn't seem to be working. The first category of medicines is antidepressants.

Antidepressants. These medications are usually preferred for those patients who are not only suffering from ADHD but also have symptoms of depression. The antidepressants that are prescribed to the patients in these cases aim at more than one neurotransmitter—the most popularly used antidepressant, in this case, Wellbutrin. Bupropion is the generic name of this medicine. This medicine aims at both dopamine and norepinephrine. Apart from this, there is another line of treatment open to the doctors, which involves the use of tricyclic antidepressants. The side effects of this medication are quite mild, but the patient might experience a loss of appetite, irritability, worsening, or Tourette's syndrome or tics, and decreased sleep.

Medications for high blood pressure. These medications are also used in the treatment of ADHD. But not all medications of this category are suitable for ADHD treatment. Some common names include guanfacine or Tenex and clonidine or Catapres. However, it has been reported that these medications do not help with increasing attention. But they are helpful in decreasing hyperactivity, aggression, and impulsivity.

When Should I Take Medications?

This is the most common question that is asked by the ADHD patients. Even though it might seem like an easy decision, it is not. Today, people are aware of a lot of facts regarding ADHD, and yet they are not enough to make this decision. Well, what I can tell you is that you shouldn't make this decision in a hurry. Think it through and take your time if you are still unsure. Judge all the options that are present in front of you. But lastly, you should never overlook your instinct. If you get a gut feeling that this is going to be good for you, go with it. If your doctor is telling you to take the medication, consider it but never let anyone pressurize you into taking certain types of meds.

If you want to have a better idea about the medications in ADHD treatment, then you should visit a specialist and clarify your queries. Some common things that you should ask are as follows –

- Is medication absolutely necessary to help me manage my symptoms?
- What are the treatment options that I have in front of me?
- What is the effectiveness of these medications?
- Considering my symptoms, what is your choice of medications for me? Do these medications have any side effects?
- During the course of the treatment, will the medications have to be taken throughout?
- How will I know when I have to stop taking the medications? What are the signs?

Remember that taking medications is not the only type of treatment approach there is for ADHD. The challenges posed by ADHD can be conquered by other methods as well, and the patient can still lead a life that is productive. Here, I am listing some common strategies that have to be used alongside the medications so that your dosage can be kept low.

- For starters, what you eat is very important. Your diet should be healthy. Your diet not only has a direct effect on your symptoms, but it can also uplift your mood and help you concentrate. If you eat the right type of food, you will find yourself with greater energy levels than before. So, have a fixed time for eating your meals and also include some snacks in your meal plan in between the major meals. Your diet should be rich in magnesium, iron, and zinc alongside the omega-3 fatty acids.

- The next thing to do is to have a regular exercise schedule. Exercising daily doesn't mean that you have to do some kind of intense workout. Any type of physical activity helps elevate the levels of serotonin, norepinephrine, and dopamine. Your ability to stay attentive and focused is affected by all of these neurochemicals. If you don't want to hit the gym, you can also try dancing, skateboarding, or simply walking. Do anything you love that involves burning some calories. Put down your mobile phone on weekends and go outside for a walk. You will automatically feel replenished.

- Give a shot at therapy. Coping with your problems can become easier with therapy. In Chapter 5, I have already explained the different types of therapy, the approaches used, and their benefits. In ADHD, there are certain habits of the patient that can flare up the symptoms, but therapy can solve this problem. There are certain therapies that are mainly focused on teaching you impulse control, and there are others that teach you how to reduce stress. You will also learn how to organize your life and manage your time. All of this will ultimately help you in achieving your goals.

- Having a good sleep at night is equally important, like everything else mentioned above. Once you start sleeping well, you will notice how drastically your symptoms are improving. Sleeping well at night is not that difficult. All you need to do is make some small changes in your sleeping habits and you will be noticing some really good changes. For starters, don't drink caffeine in the second half of the day. Also, try to set a fixed time for going to bed at night.

- Lastly, staying positive can make a massive difference in the result of the treatment. If you stay happy and positive minded, nothing can pull you down, and you will get better results.

I would also like to remind you that if you decide to start taking the medications as prescribed by your doctor, you also have to promise yourself that you are going to maintain the schedule. In order to get the effectiveness of the medications, following instructions is of utmost importance. You need to know everything about those medications, and your doctor is the best person to ask.

Also, you might not find the right medication for you in the first try. It's like a hit-and-trial method. So, you have to communicate openly and be honest in order to find the medication that suits you best.

Chapter 8: Dealing With ADHD Shame

Shame is something that lots of adult ADHD patients feel, and it can be deafening. The root cause of shame lies mostly in the fact that ADHD patients feel they have not been able to keep up others' expectations and have been a complete failure throughout their life. If not addressed, the sense of failure can hamper self-esteem and become a very big emotional burden. So, you should never be afraid to go to someone and ask them for help, especially professional help. If you are feeling sorry and perpetually unworthy, then you are also a victim of ADHD shame. It can be a haunting thing to endure for a lifetime. That is why it is of utmost importance that you find out the root cause of your shame, understand why you have to do something about it, and then take the necessary steps.

What Is Shame?

Even though it might seem unrealistic, people do misunderstand the concept of shame and mix it up with other feelings. In order to prevent, first, you must have a comprehensive idea of what shame is. If you are someone struggling with ADHD, then you already know that every day feels like you keep apologizing to others for something or the other. It might be because you didn't do the laundry, didn't clean your desk, were late to the office, or lost your car keys. No matter how hard the ADHD patients try, these things keep happening over and over again.

It eventually leads to a cycle of self-blame where apologizing for even insignificant things, becomes a habit. It happens even more in those patients who were diagnosed with ADHD later in life. Ultimately, these patients are numbed by the sense of shame, and it can be very crippling. Things can go to such an extent where people refrain from looking into their wardrobe because they know it's messy, and they are ashamed of it. They feel tortured for every disorganized part of their lives.

So, to put it in simpler terms, shame can be described as a constant state of embarrassment and feeling of inadequacy. The person feels as if he/she is humiliated all the time. In extreme cases, people are no longer the person they really are in front of others, and this gives them a feeling of having a secret life. Out of all the symptoms that ADHD patients have to face, shame is definitely one of the most painful ones, and it can easily wreak emotional havoc. The patients keep indulging in negative self-talk, and it is more or less like wearing an anvil throughout your life.

Thus, when people experience shame, they are somehow ashamed of a certain part of themselves. They struggle a lot in their daily life, but they don't want others to know about it. So, they put up a façade where they lead a happy life. But with time, this constant need to be someone else brings a feeling of loneliness, and it is exhausting. The patients start withdrawing themselves from their close ones as well, and eventually, they can't seek support from their family members because they are crippled by shame.

There are different types of shame in ADHD, and we are going to discuss them below –

- The first type of shame is where the person is simply ashamed of the fact that they have ADHD. They cannot be comfortable with this medical condition. Even though it is a lifelong condition and people have to accept it as if they have different hair colors, it is not so easy.

- The next type of shame that ADHD patients feel is that they are different from others. They look at others, and then they look at themselves. They notice significant differences. This shame of not being the same as others is more crippling in children than in adults. Everyone has the desire to fit in, but with ADHD, you will always have differences that will make you stand out in the room (and not in a good way). This constant attention that ADHD patients receive when they walk into a room also gives them social anxiety. But it is not only the behavioral differences that set them apart, ADHD patients often need extra help, and they also have to take meds throughout the day and keep up with their doctor's appointments.

- The next type of shame that ADHD patients have is about their behaviors. They do not behave the same as others. They almost always end up doing something where others make them feel embarrassed. They feel embarrassed because their work desk or their home is not as tidy and clean as that of others'. Every person is affected differently when it comes to behavioral shame. But all of them have one thing in common – they are ashamed.

- Another common type of shame noticed in ADHD adults is that they are not satisfied with their position in life, and they feel that they did not put in enough effort. They had set certain goals, and they feel like they haven't reached those milestones. The shame from this feeling is worsened when they see others around them doing great things while they can't. This also causes resentment because the ADHD adults are just as smart as the others, and yet they have drawbacks.

- ADHD patients keep ruminating about their pasts, and they bring up every instance in their minds where they failed at doing something. It can be the time they missed paying their credit card bill or the time when they had to break up with someone special. It can also be the most embarrassing moment of their life. They keep playing it over and over again, and they relive that shame from time to time.

You should also understand that shame and guilt are two very different things. You feel guilty about what you have done but you feel ashamed of who you are as a person.

Consequences of Shame

Now that you have a clear idea of what shame is let us move on to the consequences of ADHD shame. As you already know, people with ADHD face intense emotions. Whatever normal emotions they have are intensified to a great extent. And, shame can lead to some pretty nasty emotions. Here are some of the common ways in which shame can affect the lives of ADHD patients –

- People try to conceal their own personalities because they feel ashamed. They avoid any situation where they have to be emotionally vulnerable, and this impacts their relationships to a great extent. We are going to explore how ADHD impacts relationships in greater detail in the next chapter. But for now, you should know that ADHD patients shy away from friendships or even intimacy because revealing their personality and who they are, makes them feel vulnerable.

- ADHD shame makes the patients not express their emotions. They start bottling up a lot of feelings. This leads to depression. The tendency to suppress one's emotions is even more common in women as compared to men. They might be ashamed of an incident that happened to them, or they might be ashamed of the person they are. Whatever the reason is, the person keeps suppressing all his emotions and thoughts inside their heart, and this eventually leads to severe mental health conditions.

- The direct result of both the above-mentioned consequences is that the ADHD patient is pushed into a state of constant anxiety, depression, and worthlessness. Their self-esteem takes a hit and becomes impaired. Every day in their life feels like a battle that they have to endure.

- Relapse into more severe phases is more common in those ADHD patients who face shame in a more intense manner. Someone who might have overcome substance abuse might relapse back into it just because they have this crippling sense of shame at the back of their heads. In fact, there have been cases where people purposefully gave into problematic behavior just because they think healing is not possible for them. That is why it is said by specialists that very often, the reason why ADHD patients don't consider therapy or any form of treatment is because of the shame they have. They think that since they are worthless, there is no point in opting for treatment.

So, as you can see from the points mentioned above, shame pushes you into a cycle of self-rumination and negative self-talk. Sometimes people try to cease that pain by turning to alcohol or drugs, both of which make the problem worse. In extreme cases, shame takes the shape of anger, and people start becoming aggressive. Even when their loved ones try to help them out, they push everyone away. If you are a family member of an ADHD patient reading this book, then I would urge you to understand that when the patient is pushing you away, that is when they need you the most. They simply don't see it, and so, you cannot give up on them.

How to Silence the Haters?

One of the main sources of ADHD shame is the haters in the society who don't know anything about the disorder and yet, treat it as an untouchable thing. The reason behind this is the several misconceptions that are present in society. But if you want to deal with ADHD shame and not let it control you, then you have to silence the skeptics, and we are going to talk about it in this section.

Very often, you will find that skeptics make it absolutely clear that adults cannot have ADHD and that they are simply using it as an excuse to cover up their faults. They keep saying that whatever symptoms they are having or claim to have is because their parents did not hold the reins when they were young. They will tell you to deal with your shortcomings and grow up. But I have already given you plenty of evidence in this book to support the fact that ADHD is real. It is very real, and it happens in adults as well. So, if you do have to reply to the skeptics, do so with facts. One of the best ammunition you can produce in front of the skeptics of society is a hard fact. You can even take him/her to one of your meetings with your support group or send them articles that will educate them.

But if you are looking for something sarcastic, you can always tell them how nice it is for them to be smarter than some of the most renowned psychologists and scientists in the world.

Then comes another group of people who are best described as the crusaders. They will question every step you take and every decision you make. They will second guess your choice of doctor or even your medication. They might even tell you that ADHD medications are nothing but 'kiddie cocaine,' but then, you have to present them with facts that, like every other medication, ADHD meds have their side-effects too. But that does not mean they are going to inculcate a feeling of dependency in the patient. Before you go spouting off things to others, you need to make sure you have your facts straight. So, read as many articles as you can so that you can make an informed speech about how drug therapy is actually important for ADHD patients.

At the end of the day, you have to let go of others think of you. You need to focus on yourself and your decisions. Ask yourself – do you want to take medications? Do medications make you feel better? Are you comfortable with taking medications? If the answer to these questions is yes, then who cares what others think? So, the next time someone comes to you with their holier than thou attitude about drug therapy, you can simply ask them would they deny taking insulin if they had been diagnosed with diabetes?

Then there are some people who like to make sarcastic jokes about ADHD symptoms. They might say things like 'If only I had ADHD, I could come up with some excuse for forgetting deadlines every month.' When you protest, saying that these comments are disrespectful, they might say they were simply joking. The best way to deal with such people is to ignore them and not respond until the right moment comes. For example, if it is your boss who keeps humiliating you for your ADHD, you should avoid responding to those comments. Start looking for a new job, and when you find one, you can write a detailed report to the main office stating how your boss abused you just because of a medical condition. If you think you cannot put up with it any longer, you can use the direct approach and see how your boss responds. You can tell them that these comments are hurtful, and you'd like him not to continue being sarcastic. If this works, then it is okay; if it doesn't, then you have to wait for the right time to submit a written complaint.

The next type of people are the ones closest to us and yet fail to understand that ADHD is a real problem. No matter how much evidence you provide them, they will not believe you. They might keep telling you that there is nothing wrong with you, and you are simply being lazy. Experts believe that family members often behave in such a manner because of the fact that they cannot accept that anything like ADHD exists. Moreover, they cannot accept that it might run in their family, so they go into denial. So, if you have someone like that in your family, you have to stand up to them and let them know that ADHD is a condition that you are suffering from, and it is not about them. In the beginning, it might be difficult, but as time passes, these types of people will give up.

How to Heal Shame?

No matter how you reply to the haters of the society, the shame lingers on, and you have to figure out a way to heal yourself. No matter how much qualified a person becomes in life if they feel ashamed because of ADHD, no degree or educational qualification can reduce it. Eliminating shame is something that is not possible for everyone. There is some amount of shame in all of us but what you can do is reduce the toxic levels of shame, and here are some tips on how you can do it –

- **Educate yourself** – The first step is to obviously educate yourself about ADHD so that you don't have any misconceptions. Understand that all the behaviors and traits that you have are because of some genetic and neurobiological reasons. It is not about your character, and so there is nothing wrong with you. It is not your fault, and you have to understand that. Different areas of life are hampered because of ADHD, and you are not the only one here. It happens to every patient. Go back to the first two chapters of this book and remind yourself that ADHD is a biological condition. When you educate yourself more and more, it will become easier for you to acknowledge th fact that ADHD is, in fact, a neurological condition. You will realize that many of the causes of your shame are nothing but a result of your ADHD. With time, you will see how the majority of shame was self-inflicted.

- **Have your own support system** – If you don't have people supporting you in your journey to fight ADHD, then you need to build one right now. It can be a local support group where you go for meetings, meet similar people, and share your experiences. Or, it can also be your therapist or any family member who truly understand you and supports you. When you connect with people who understand the problem, you will feel heard. If you have a busy lifestyle and you think that you cannot make time for support groups in your locality, you can also search for online support groups. Some of them even conduct webinars from time to time.

- **Change your mindset** – Pay careful attention to how you think of yourself or how you talk to people when you have to talk about yourself. Do you talk too much in negatives? Do you say things like 'I am never going to become good at managing time'? If yes, then it is time you change these things. You should say that 'I know it is difficult, but I can slowly learn how to manage my time'. Such sentences promote hope and motivation. Several people think that bringing a shift in your mindset is about neglecting the problem. But that is not the case – you have to change yourself to a positive person where you are open to all possibilities. You will let go of your limiting beliefs. You will stop judging yourself and start believing that it is okay to make mistakes but what is important is that you are ready to fix them.

Practice Self-Love

Loving yourself can be really helpful in overcoming ADHD shame. You may find it strange and difficult in the beginning because you are used to blaming yourself for every small thing and being ashamed of who you are. Put yourself first and look out for your happiness and well-being. This will surely help you to heal from shame. Let us discuss some of the self-love practices that you can do to become a fully functioning and self-sufficient individual who can take care of themselves and live a happy life.

Take Help From Others
If you love yourself, never hesitate to ask for help and to receive help. We are social creatures, and we constantly need each other to survive. When you are overwhelmed, anxious, confused, or lonely, make sure that you reach out to people instead of sinking in your own grief and shame. Sometimes a good company can provide you guidance and comfort. If you let your grief and emotions get the best of you, then you will not be able to calm yourself or think. People think that asking for help is what weak people do, but it is not like that. If you help others at their difficult times, then you deserve to get helped in your crisis as well. When your problems are serious and persistent, go to your friends, family, or someone professional like a therapist.

Meet Your Own Needs
Pay attention to yourself and cater to your needs. If you keep on worrying about meeting the needs of others and neglect your own needs and concerns, then you will end up nowhere. It is high time that you stop all these things and start putting yourself first. In case you are habituated with someone else taking care of all your needs, then you need to stop that as well.

With ADHD, it can be difficult, but doing some things on your own will make you feel better. Make sure that you meet the basic physical needs like a dental checkup, medical checkup, exercise, rest, food, etc. Give a little extra attention to those needs and requirements which you are most likely to overlook. When you feel tired, confused, overwhelmed, afraid, angry, sad, lonely, or victimized, try asking yourself what will comfort you and go for it straight away. The reason for your depression may also be the fact that you have been neglecting and avoiding yourself for a prolonged time.

Start Having Fun
Start planning hobbies, recreation, and pleasures. If you keep on focusing on the gloomy side of your life and constantly stay overwhelmed with your problems, your life will become a competition or a struggle of achievement and endurance. Life should not be a burden, so don't go too hard on yourself. Sometimes, a little bit of enjoyment and laughter is all you need to get back on track.

Protect Yourself
Protecting yourself from mental, emotional, and physical abuse is an essential part of self-love. If you love someone, then that doesn't mean that you have to accept mean and insulting behaviors from them. If you think that you are abused or violated, stop wasting your energy and time in expecting to change that person. Take a stand for yourself and cut them off your life. In the section 'How to Silence the Haters?' I

have explained some of the ways you can stand up for yourself. But if situations arise that are not mentioned, be creative and deal with the haters with a stern hand. Never blame yourself for the hate spewed upon you by others.

Be Gentle to Yourself
Treat yourself with compassion and gentleness. Make your inner voice a little kind and calm towards yourself. When you are in pain or any kind of crisis, blaming yourself will not do any good. It will just make things harder and worse for you. And when you have ADHD, these feelings manifest themselves more intensely. In situations like these, you may be tempted to distract yourself and ignore your feelings, but make sure that you don't do that. Instead, just try to be with yourself. You are the one who should be with yourself the most when you are in fear, anger, hopelessness, sorrow, or anxiety. The innocent child inside of you needs you the most. Try to comfort yourself with compassion, kindness, and tenderness, just the way you do for others. Listen to yourself and start forgiving yourself. Embrace yourself and build trust in yourself. Never give up on yourself.

Start Accepting Yourself
Loving and accepting yourself includes your shortcomings, thoughts, feelings, and appearance. You don't need to prove anything to anybody. You deserve respect and love, regardless of all your flaws. Others will always try to search for opportunities to violate your flaws and weaknesses. Stop seeking

validation from others and accept your own flaws and weaknesses. In this way, you can prevent yourself from getting violated by others and become a spontaneous and authentic person.

Encourage Yourself
Treat yourself with enthusiasm and encouragement. There should be a positive coach inside you who will always encourage you to do things you love. Don't wait for others to give you compliments or appreciation. Give credit for what you are good at, instead of taking those for granted. Encourage yourself to make even the slightest progress towards your dreams and aspirations.

Express Yourself
Don't keep your inner self hidden for too long. Start honoring yourself and communicate your needs, thoughts, opinions, and feelings. Always remember that you have a right to have an opinion that is different from others. You are unique, and you can feel and state whatever you want without owing a justification to anybody. If you start stating your opinions fearlessly, you will start earning other's respect as well. Don't worry about the fact that you have ADHD. Does having diabetes mean that you won't voice your thoughts? No, right? The same goes for ADHD.

Start Having a Spiritual Practice
Start to spend more time with yourself. Regardless of your belief in God, spiritual practice will really help

you to create a deep relationship with yourself. Having some quiet time for your self is a great way of honoring yourself. Religious beliefs are not necessarily required for spiritual practice. By doing this, you can find a place that is calm and centered from where you can access inner guidance for experiencing harmony with others and yourself. When you invest more time in listening to yourself and in finding the truth for yourself, you get peace, clarity, and confidence. It will help you to keep your calm and your mind in the right state no matter what happens around you. In Chapter 3, we have elaborated on the concept of mindfulness meditation.

Lastly, I would like to say that you should go to a therapist who is experienced in working with ADHD patients struggling with shame. Learn to be compassionate because you deserve that. Treat your body in a positive light and yourself as a child. Take care of yourself as a child, and you will see what an incredible difference it can have on your body and mind. You can even prepare a checklist of all things (big and small) that you can do to decrease your sense of shame. The more you let shame take hold of you, the more you will give in to the lies of the society. Have faith in yourself. The path might not be easy, but you have it in yourself to walk upon it.

Chapter 9: ADHD and Relationships

In this chapter, we are solely going to focus on how the different relationships in our lives are affected by ADHD. It is true that it can lead to resentments, frustrations, and several misunderstandings. You will even push away the people who are closest to you. But on the brighter side, there different strategies that you can follow to mend these relationships and lead a happy life.

What Is the Impact of ADHD on Relationships?

The usual symptoms of impulsivity and hypersensitivity can wreak havoc in different areas of your life, but they can also cause a dent in your personal relationships. It can become worse for those who have not yet been diagnosed with ADHD or are not receiving proper treatment.

First, let us see what impact ADHD has on your life if you are the one suffering from ADHD.

- As you might already know, one of the most common symptoms of ADHD is being distracted at all times. But when it comes to relationships, being distracted can cause a lot of problems. Your partner might think that you are neglecting them. Staying distracted at all times might also lead you to not keep up on important promises that you have made. Gradually, your partner will start feeling unwanted and unheard. You might love your partner way too much, but because of the symptoms of ADHD, if you don't show your love for your partner, he/she will start feeling like they have been left alone.

- The next thing that I want to mention is being hyperfocused. This is a tendency noticed in ADHD patients. Sometimes they become so hyperfocused at something that they forget everything in their surroundings. It is somewhat exactly opposite to what distractibility is. Your loved one might start feeling left out or unimportant because you can't seem to drag yourself away from the thing that you are hyperfocused on.

- Next, let's talk about forgetfulness and how it impacts relationships. I don't think I have to emphasize much on how partners might feel if you forget important dates or a dinner date that you were supposed to attend after your meeting. Your husband might feel that you left him stranded just for nothing. You might forget your share of the responsibilities from time to time, like cleaning the house, paying the bills, and so on. Eventually, your partner will feel like they cannot rely on you for even such basic tasks, let alone anything important. In this way, resentment keeps building on both sides.

- We all know that ADHD patients struggle with being organized. They might leave their tasks without finishing them or keep piles of stuff lying here and there. This can be a problem if you are in a relationship with someone who prefers things to be kept tidy and clean. So, you being disorganized is not only stressful for you but also for them. And so, this is what gives birth to constant nagging in relationships with an ADHD person.

- Another very prominent trait of ADHD people is their impulsivity. This can be problematic in relationships. Impulsiveness will prompt you to act before thinking anything through. One very common example of this problem is when you keep spending money without any reason and just because you felt like it. This often results in credit cards being maxed out and too many things in the house, causing a shortage of space. However, there are some ADHD patients who show some more dangerous symptoms of impulsivity – they love to drive recklessly or love to have risky sex. They might even prefer using inappropriate words in public places. All of these things lead to compatibility issues among partners.

- Procrastination in ADHD patients can also affect relationships. For example, whenever you are on tight deadlines because you procrastinated all along, you might be extra fussy and irritated at your partner without proper reason. No one likes to be treated that way, and so this is another reason for disputes in close relationships with ADHD patients.

- Lastly, ADHD patients have terrible mood swings from time to time. At one moment, they are happy, and the next moment, they are terribly angry at some incident, which is insignificant. This leads to frustration and anxiety, both of which can take away the happiness of your relationships. Your partner might constantly feel on edge and this is not good if you want your relationship to be stable.

Now, if you are the person who is in a relationship with someone having ADHD, you will constantly feel that you are unappreciated, ignored, and lonely. You will find your partner not keeping any of the promises they made or not remembering things you wanted them to remember. In fact, you might even feel that the person you love so much doesn't even care about the relationship.

So, now that you have seen how both parties in a relationship are affected, you can understand how destructive it is. But you can fix it and get out of this toxic cycle. Read on to find out how.

Tips for a Healthier Relationship

If you want to turn your relationship into a healthier one, then here are some tips that you should follow –

- **Walk in your partner's shoes** – The first step to mending a broken relationship is to understand your partner. You have to place yourself in their position and then understand their perspective of things. But you also have to keep in mind that it is extremely easy to misunderstand and misinterpret things. If you have ADHD and your partner doesn't, then you have to understand that there are a lot of differences between you both and how you think. So, if you truly want to understand your partner, it's best if you go and ask them.

- **Learn about ADHD** – In order to mend your relationship, you have to know everything there is to know about ADHD. You will understand its influence on you and your partner once you know about the symptoms and why they happen. If your partner doesn't have ADHD, but you are the one who has it, then it is all the more important for your partner to learn about this disorder. Then, it will become easier for him/her to understand your actions.

- **Acknowledge that you need to work on your relationship** – Many a time, relationships falter because the partners fail to notice or rather don't want to acknowledge that their relationship needs work. Constant criticism and nagging are not going to get you anywhere. If you cannot figure out a way yourself, then you should seek professional help and opt for a couple's counseling from a specialist who has experience in dealing with ADHD patients.

- **Take responsibility** – Being responsible for your actions is very important not only for the partner who has ADHD but also for the one who doesn't. You can make progress in your relationship only when you own up to your actions. It is true that the symptoms of ADHD itself cause a lot of problems, but it is not right to put all the blame on the disorder alone. The partner is also at fault. No matter what your symptoms are, it is in your hands how you choose to react to a particular situation. It is your reaction that will determine whether your partner feels loved or ignored.

Now, there are some things I would like to say to the non-ADHD partner because even you have certain responsibilities to take care of. You have to understand what your partner is going through. ADHD can make a person feel constantly guilty and ashamed, and stressed. They are overwhelmed by the simplest things in life. So, if you notice that your partner is experiencing some strong emotions, ask them to take a time out, and then you can talk it through after a while. Acknowledge the fact that it is not always your partner's fault. They are not always unreasonable. Sometimes it is their symptoms acting up. Care for your partner just the way you want them to care for you. Finally, look for ways in which the symptoms of your partner can be managed because once that happens, your relationship will start getting better as well.

Conclusion

Thank you for making it through to the end of *ADHD Workbook for Adults*; let us hope that you were able to get answers to all the questions you had in mind. I hope you have gained some knowledge from the insight that I shared in this book. Each and every strategy that has been mentioned in this book has been proven to bring the symptoms of ADHD under control and make your life easier.

The next step is to apply these strategies in your life so that you can lead a more fulfilled life with your loved ones. I understand that it is not always easy to deal with the symptoms of ADHD every day. It takes a lot of courage to tackle your issues head-on and put in all the hard work that is required to overcome the problems. It is quite probable that the first medicate you take, or the first therapy you seek might not work for you. But don't let that one moment discourage you from the path of seeking treatment because the right treatment is out there; you simply have to find it. There might be several instances where you have to try medications that are not the right fit for you, but only after you try things you will come to know what works for you and what doesn't. I had personally known so many people who had had to try several therapies and medications before they finally got 'the one' they had been looking for. The idea is to never lose hope.

Every journey has its own setbacks, and yours is no different. But there is no need to beat yourself up for a couple of failures. You need to keep reminding yourself to stay strong. Love yourself and give yourself a pat on the back whenever you make the least progress. Tell yourself that every challenge that comes on your path is just another opportunity for you to grow as a human being and learn new things along the way.

The one advice that I give to everyone is that if you want success in your battle against ADHD, you first have to learn how to accept yourself. No matter how many failures you receive, you have to stay excited and motivated for the new opportunities to come. Whenever you are starting to walk on a new path, it is always better that you start with a note of positivity. A positive mind will take you places. Just because you have ADHD doesn't mean that you cannot have a balanced life. You simply have to learn how you can work together with other people and improve your communication skills. If things seem too much to handle on your own, learn to delegate because it is always better to take help from others than do a task all by yourself and ruin it.

You will notice that organization is not your strongest skill set, but you have to come up with something practical that you can follow in your life. Take help from your close people or your family members whom you trust. Think about how you can come up with a system of planning things that will be easier to memorize and not much of a hassle. The moment you come up with a routine, your life will seem less chaotic because now, you have a set of tasks to complete within certain time frames. You should even plan your sleep and your meals so that you don't forget anything.

Agreeing to do too many things at a time can cause a lot of trouble in your life. But your tendency to become impulsive will force you to indulge in such behaviors. That is why it is important for every ADHD patient to learn to say no. The more work you take, the more jam-packed your routine is going to become, leaving you stresses and overwhelmed. Your ability to lead a lifestyle that is healthy depends largely on how well you prioritize your work and other commitments. So, whenever someone presents you with a new opportunity, take a moment to check your schedule and see how much you already have on your plate.

Don't pay heed to any of the ADHD myths or rumors in your surroundings. If you want to know something about ADHD, always read articles from trustworthy pages. Don't let anyone make you feel that you are lazy or using ADHD as an excuse. ADHD is a very real problem, and it is a disorder. Choose your therapist wisely because he/she is going to help you a lot in managing your symptoms.

There are so many challenges that ADHD patients have to face in their day-to-day life. From organizational difficulties to problems in time management, they have to put in more effort than others even when they are doing the simplest tasks. ADHD patients who already have a challenging job to handle find it even more difficult because it is no easy task. But take it one step at a time. Don't try to change everything all at once because that will only leave you even more overwhelmed. No matter what you do, don't overlook the stress that you are taking upon yourself. Keep a check on the stress levels. Engage in some physical activity even if it means going for a stroll in the neighborhood and eat a healthy diet. Practicing these healthy habits will also benefit you in the long-term by reducing your symptoms. Slowly, you will see how manageable your life becomes. Lastly, I would also encourage you to practice mindfulness and yoga, both of which will help in calming your mind. It will also help you exercise greater control over yourself and your emotions. If you are just a beginner, meditate for a shorter time span, and then you can gradually increase it.

I hope that the treatment options and the tips that I had mentioned in this book have come of help to you. If you doubt that you have been suffering from this disorder, then you should not be wasting any more time and meet the doctor at once. The longer you take to seek professional help, the more your condition will deteriorate. The right treatment is out there in front of you, and all you need to do is ask for it.

Finally, I would highly appreciate it if you can leave a review on Amazon if this book has helped you in any manner.

Resources

Alexander T. Vazsonyi, J. M. (2017). It's time: A meta-analysis on the self-control-deviance link. *Journal of Criminal Justice, 48*, 48-63.

Amelia Villagomez, U. R. (2014). Iron, Magnesium, Vitamin D, and Zinc Deficiencies in Children Presenting with Symptoms of Attention-Deficit/Hyperactivity Disorder. *Children, 1*(3), 261-279.

Anne Halmøy, O. B. (2009). Occupational Outcome in Adult ADHD: Impact of Symptom Profile, Comorbid Psychiatric Problems, and Treatment. *Journal of Attention Disorders, 13*(2), 175-187.

Aparajita B. Kuriyan, W. E. (2012). Young Adult Educational and Vocational Outcomes of Children Diagnosed with ADHD. *Journal of Abnormal Child Psychology, 41*(1), 27-41.

Benjamín Piñeiro-Dieguez, V. B.-M.-G.-L. (2016). Psychiatric Comorbidity at the Time of Diagnosis in Adults With ADHD. *Journal of Attention Disorders, 20*(12), 1066-1075.

Joel T. Nigg, K. L. (2012). Meta-Analysis of Attention-Deficit/Hyperactivity Disorder or Attention-Deficit/Hyperactivity Disorder Symptoms, Restriction Diet, and Synthetic Food Color Additives. *Journal of the American Academy of Child & Adolescent Psychiatry, 51*(1), 86-97.

John T. Mitchell, L. Z. (2015). Mindfulness Meditation Training for Attention-

Deficit/Hyperactivity Disorder in Adulthood: Current Empirical Support, Treatment Overview, and Future Directions. *Cognitive and Behavioral Practice, 22*(2), 172-191.

L. Eugene Arnold, N. L. (2012). Artificial Food Colors and Attention-Deficit/Hyperactivity Symptoms: Conclusions to Dye for. *Neurotherapeutics, 9*(3), 599-609.

Michael H. Bloch, J. M. (2014). Nutritional Supplements for the Treatment of ADHD. *Child and Adolescent Psychiatric Clinics of North America, 23*(4), 883-897.

Rucklidge, J. J. (2010). Gender Differences in Attention-Deficit/Hyperactivity Disorder. *Psychiatric Clinics of North America, 33*(2), 357-373.

Saskia van der Oord, S. M. (2011). The Effectiveness of Mindfulness Training for Children with ADHD and Mindful Parenting for their Parents. *Journal of Child and Family Studies, 21*(1), 139-147.

Stéphanie Baggio, A. F. (2018). Prevalence of Attention Deficit Hyperactivity Disorder in Detention Settings: A Systematic Review and Meta-Analysis. *Frontiers in Psychiatry, 9*.

Stephen P. Hinshaw, E. B.-N. (2012). Prospective follow-up of girls with attention-deficit/hyperactivity disorder into early adulthood: Continuing impairment includes elevated risk for suicide attempts and self-injury. *Journal of Consulting and Clinical Psychology, 80*(6), 1041-1051.

Winston Chung, S.-F. J. (2019). Trends in the Prevalence and Incidence of Attention-Deficit/Hyperactivity Disorder Among Adults and Children of Different Racial and Ethnic Groups. *JAMA Network Open, 2*(11).

Ylva Ginsberg, J. Q. (2014). Underdiagnosis of Attention-Deficit/Hyperactivity Disorder in Adult Patients. *The Primary Care Companion For CNS Disorders.*

Zheng Chang, P. D. (2017). Association Between Medication Use for Attention-Deficit/Hyperactivity Disorder and Risk of Motor Vehicle Crashes. *JAMA Psychiatry, 74*(6), 597.

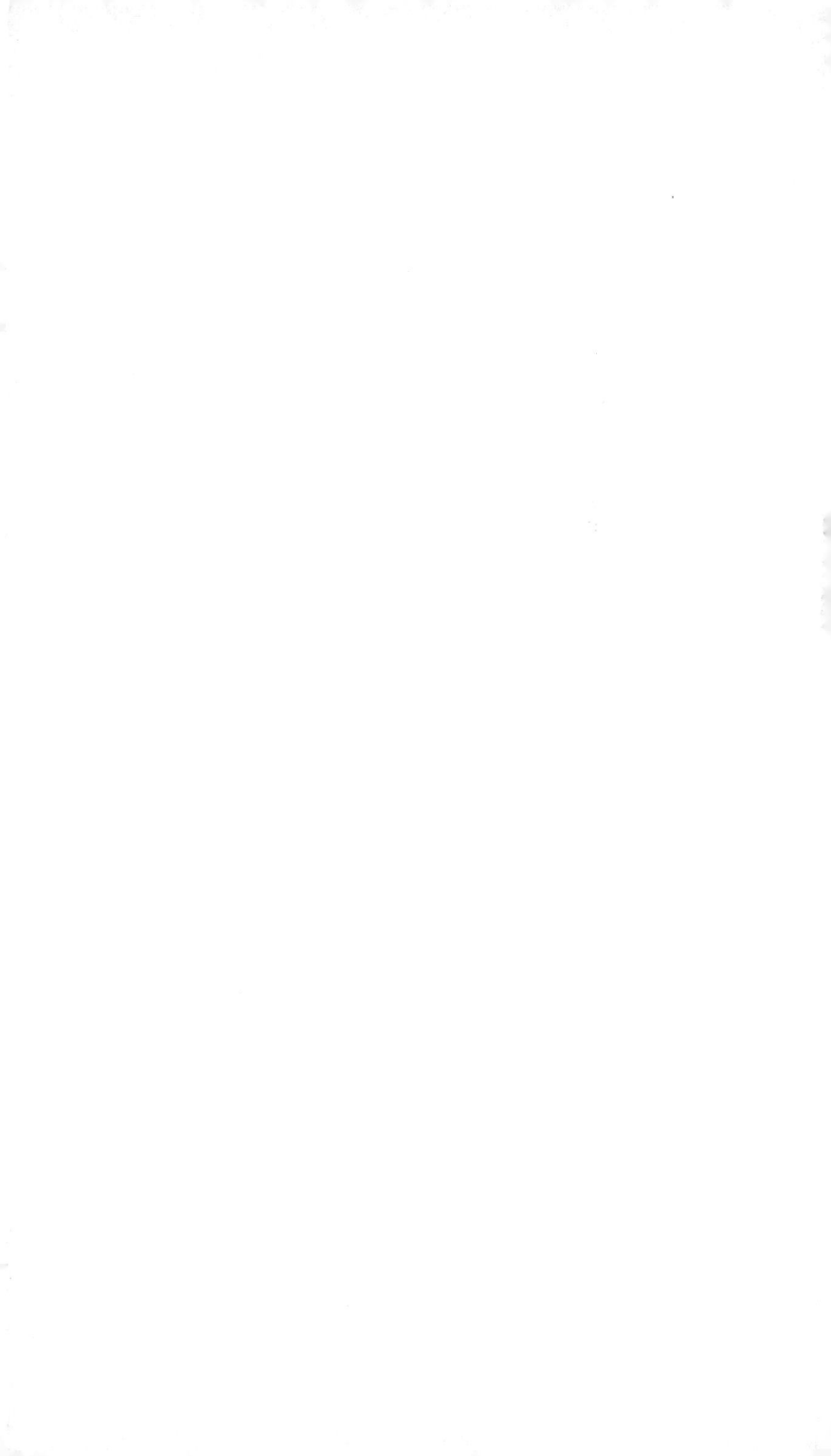

Printed in Great Britain
by Amazon